After leaving Oxford University with a Modern Languages degree, Barbara Paterson worked as an advertising copywriter. She later turned freelance in an effort to juggle work and domestic responsibilities. After being intermittently a translator, teacher, market researcher and tourist guide, she concentrated on editorial writing. Apart from books, she wrote many articles and short stories under her own name and various pseudonyms. Her interest in food and chemical allergies began as a result of her personal experiences: three years' research culminating in THE ALLERGY CONNECTION (Thorsons, 1985).

She was married to a New Zealander – also a writer – and lived in West London all her adult life. Of their three children, two are writers and the third has more sense.

She died, of cancer, in June 1986.

The 'A' for Allergy
Diet Book

Barbara Paterson

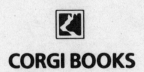

CORGI BOOKS

THE 'A' FOR ALLERGY DIET BOOK

A CORGI BOOK   0 552 12829 5

First publication in Great Britain

PRINTING HISTORY
Corgi edition published 1986

Copyright © Barbara Paterson 1986

This book is set in 10/11 pt Plantin Compugraphic by Colset
Private Limited, Singapore.

Corgi Books are published by Transworld Publishers Ltd.,
61–63 Uxbridge Road, Ealing, London W5 5SA, in Australia
by Transworld Publishers (Aust.) Pty. Ltd., 15–23 Helles
Avenue, Moorebank, NSW 2170, and in New Zealand by
Transworld Publishers (N.Z.) Ltd., Cnr. Moselle and
Waipareira Avenues, Henderson, Auckland.

Made and printed in Great Britain by
Cox & Wyman Ltd., Reading, Berks.

To all the doctors and patients who were ready to give up their time and to share their knowledge and experience

Thank you

'When people stop eating the
things that are wrong for them,
the fat melts away like butter in the sun'
                                    Dr E.H.

Contents

CHAPTER 1

PEOPLE LIKE YOU?

**'Now I come out from behind the counter to greet customers'
Jill C, 38, explains how her weight problems disappeared
(and her personality changed dramatically) after discovering
her own allergy-free diet**

For years and years I was obsessed with my weight. It was the
single most important thing in my life. Ridiculous really.

I've even been through the whole psychological bit. Eighteen
months ago I was sent to psychiatrists. They delved deep into my
whole family background and history – I was tied up in knots. They
ended by almost making me believe that I'd had some sort of deprived
childhood. I went faithfully every week for six months, but by the
time I stopped going I was still binge-eating.

Thinking back to my childhood, I can see how the pattern started. I
was always nibbling. Pick pick picking. While I was doing the wash-
ing-up I'd be helping myself to little bits of this and that. And my
Dad's overweight. We'd joke about it – call him The Square Man:
5 ft high by 5 ft wide!

As long as I remember I've been overweight. Always withdrawn. I
never had any self-confidence. I was very heavy by the time I was
fifteen; I weighed 11 stone. They sent me to hospital to see a specialist.
He gave me a horrible internal examination. I've never forgotten
it – it was dreadful. Then all he said was: 'Her trouble is: she's fat.'
What a thing to say to a fifteen-year-old. I'd even less confidence after
that.

When I was seventeen I started dieting. It was the sort of diet that
was popular then: four biscuits and a glass of milk and nothing else.
I'd stick to it faithfully for days at a time, and in fact I did lose weight.
Then I'd snap and I'd binge. Always the same way. I'd start with
bread and then biscuits. Then ice cream, and after that just about
anything I could lay my hands on.

I'd never done that before in my life. Although I'd been overweight, I'd never been hung up on food. The binge-eating started
along with the so-called diet.

As I grew older, it dawned on me that all this wasn't a good idea. So instead of dieting I'd take three laxatives at night, two or three times a week.

I married at nineteen. Oddly enough, it didn't do anything for my confidence. I just felt very lucky. I didn't feel I deserved anything. My husband's a smasher, but I kept on thinking: Why ever does he want me? Until the past three months all my married life has been wasted, worrying and worrying about my weight. He's put up with that all these years.

I began to go the round of the slimming clubs. I don't want to knock them at all. I know they're right for a lot of people, but they weren't right for me. Of course I can see now why not.

I got to my Gold Weight with Weight-Watchers and I got to my Gold Weight with Silhouette. But even those times when I did lose weight I still felt a fat person inside. And the weight always went back on again.

My problem was that I just couldn't stick to their diets permanently. Weight-Watchers divide foods into 'good' foods and 'bad' foods, and of course the good foods *are* good foods for most people: fish and meat and plenty of fruit and vegetables.

But naturally they do allow some bread, and I know now that bread triggers me off. And I used to keep a bowl of 'goodies' in the fridge – raw carrots and apples and so on – so I wouldn't be tempted into eating 'baddies'. I thought I was doing the right thing, but I know now that I'm allergic to both of them. I'd eat cheese and ham three or four times a week, and I know now that I shouldn't eat either of them at all.

It was amazing how my weight could change. Once at Weight-Watchers they could hardly believe it: I'd gained 10½ lbs in one week! But I lost it all the following week. That wasn't the only time, but it's the one I remember most clearly.

The trouble always was that sooner or later I'd binge-eat. If I had one slice of bread extra I couldn't stop. I'd just go on and on. Sometimes I couldn't stop eating for days. It sounds dreadful, but I'd wake up in the morning and plan my eating day. I could literally put on 7 lbs in 24 hours. My legs would swell up and hang over my shoes. If I carried on, my fingers and face would blow out too.

Every night would end with me saying: Tomorrow I'll be good. And the chances were that next day I'd be bad. It was all 'good' and 'bad'. Every time I stopped to chat to a fellow Weight-Watcher she'd always end by saying 'Be good!'

Then one day I saw someone I'd met through Weight-Watchers,

and she told me how she'd been to see this doctor who had a completely different approach.

And that's how everything came to change, just three months ago.

The first thing that happened when I came to see Dr H was that he put me on the Stone Age diet.* When I reintroduced foods I found that I was allergic to wheat and cheese. Then, since I was still reacting, I went on to test other things and found that I was also allergic to some fruits and vegetables – apples, tomatoes, carrots, bananas and cauliflower – and also, as I said, to ham.

Since then I've been eating quite differently. I eat as much as I want, when I want it. Beef and chicken, fish, vegetables and fruit – the ones I'm allowed – but I haven't been counting at all. I don't get hungry. I eat regularly – I feel if I went too long without food I might not know when to start or when to stop. I feel I could go on past the point when I'm comfortably full.

It's only in the past weeks that I've come to recognise that I no longer want to eat out of control. I'm down to 9 stone from 10 stone 4. The main thing for me is that I've completely lost my obsession with weight. I used to be on and off the scales all day long. Now my actual weight in figures has lost its importance. In fact, I'm still not as light as I was sometimes in my dieting days, but I feel quite different.

I used to have spells of deep depression. I went to my GP several times, and he did his best. It was he who got me referred to the psychiatrist – he didn't know what else he could do.

It didn't help that along with the weight problems I'd developed a bad skin. It was clear as a teenager, but it gradually got worse and worse. At thirty I was told it was acne! And over the years I had various other things going wrong. The last one was a hiatus hernia, just a year ago. That's gone too now, and though I've still got a few spots here and there they're getting fewer all the time.

I am another person altogether. My family and friends and the people I meet all say the same – that it's like talking to two different people. I used to be very timid. I'd even been known to agree with people simply because I thought it had to be me who was wrong. Now I think I'm entitled to my own opinions.

I can still be tempted by foods – particularly by bread. Sometimes I still go for it. The difference is that now I don't go on. I accept the fact that it's given me a headache, but I *don't* go on to the depression stage. I accept that I've eaten the bread and that's why I've got the headache. And then I stop.

*see p. 136.

9

While when I was with Weight-Watchers I could eat one of their meals and then go on and empty the cupboard. It's not that I was really hungry. My eyes wanted the food more than my stomach. Now I don't get hunger cravings at all. I just eat more of the things I can eat.

Most of all my legs used to bother me. Even when I hadn't been bingeing I was always aware of them, always ashamed of them. Now – well, they're still on the big side, but I'm just not bothered any more. We have our own business and post office, and I've recently started working again.

Before I saw Dr H, I'd always make sure I stayed on our side of the counter. Now, I come out from behind, and I talk to our customers. I wouldn't have believed it was possible.

THREE CASE HISTORIES

'Now my problem is – I'll have to get all new clothes!'
Thomas B. 47

Thomas B. had been overweight for most of his adult life. He had also suffered from severe bronchitis ('or asthma – the doctors never seemed sure') for years. Though he had seen numerous specialists, none had been able to help.

Eventually, fearing that he would become so incapacitated that he would no longer be able to work, he consulted Dr K. 'I can admit now I was sceptical, but at the time I was willing to try anything. It was the first time ever that anyone had suggested the possibility of allergies.'

In the first nine weeks after discovering he was allergic to milk, beef, pork, wheat, citrus fruit and diesel fumes, he lost 2 stone. He was also completely clear of asthma for the first time in ten years.

'Thin as a rail'
Jessica L., 36

Jessica weighed only 6 st. 7 lbs when she came to consult Dr M. Although 'thin as a rail', she was found to be neither anaemic nor jaundiced. Nevertheless, she 'looked as though a puff of wind could blow her away'. As a child, she had suffered from constant sore throats, chesty colds and colic. In her teens, in addition to further sore throats, she began to suffer also from hayfever and conjunc-

10

tivitis. In her twenties, she experienced multiple heart problems.

Dr M diagnosed that she was allergic to a whole range of foods, and also severely affected by inhaled chemicals. She went on to a rotated diet* of safe foods, and also modified her house to reduce her exposure to chemicals.**

In two months she gained 1 stone, and went on to gain a further ½ stone. All her other symptoms disappeared. She is now 8 stone 3 lbs and has remained well ever since.

'My family are delighted. They say I was positively gaunt before, and now I look really blooming.'

'A changed child'
Simon A., 12

Simon's problems started when he was six. Not only was he large for his age, but he suffered from both asthma and hayfever. He continued to put on weight, and became increasingly disruptive at school. He lacked concentration, was unnaturally over-active, and aggressive to his fellow- pupils.

By the age of 11 – at the height of 4' 10" – he already weighed 7 stone. In addition, his behaviour had become so intolerable that he was on the verge of being admitted to a psychiatric unit.

On being put on the Stone Age diet he lost a stone in six days. The chief culprits in his case turned out to be wholemeal bread, turkey, oats, beet sugar and bananas.

Since then he has kept a stable weight, remains almost entirely symptom-free, and has become 'a changed child' both at school and at home. 'A pleasure to have around – cheerful and co-operative'.

SHORT SHORT STORIES

Brenda F, 36: 'I put on a lot of weight after my daughter's birth, from 9 stone to 11. I never seemed to be able to lose it. I suffered from constant headaches and was severely depressed. After I found I was allergic to grains, and stopped eating them, my weight dropped down to 9 stone 5 lbs and stayed there. At the same time my depression and the headaches vanished completely.'

*see p. 67
**see p. 198

11

Frances H, 39: 'After the birth of my first child I put on 2 stone very quickly and slept non-stop. Later, I became very ill, with depression and severe bladder problems. I dropped down to 7½ stone. I was nothing but a skeleton. After being found allergic to wheat, eggs, tea, cheese, mould and chemical fumes, I lost all my symptoms. Now that I'm only eating things that agree with me, I'm up to 9½ stone – the right weight for me – and I'm 100% well.'

Sheila A, 41: 'Now I am absolutely fine. My only problem – and most people would say it wasn't a problem at all! – is that my weight dropped to 8 stone 7, and it stays there. I wouldn't mind putting on another couple of pounds, but as long as I keep to my diet my weight never changes.'

Nina R, 64: 'As I grew older and gradually began to put on more weight, the arthritis I'd had since a child began to get worse too. After I went on the Stone Age diet my weight dropped from 11 stone to 9½ stone – and the arthritis disappeared so completely I actually went on a 2½ mile Fun Run!'

Sarah H, 47: 'I used to sleep the days away – always exhausted. My weight went up to 18 stone – when I used to weigh around nine. I had a terrible cough that never left me, a permanently leaky bladder, and terrible depression. After being found allergic to wheat, sugar, butter, creosote and other chemical fumes, within months I had changed completely. My weight dropped right back down again. I feel marvellous.'

CHAPTER 2

WHEN WEIGHT PROBLEMS = FOOD ALLERGY

Of course you're not a mirror image of a Jill, or a Thomas, or a Jessica; but if something in their stories - or in any of the others' - rang a bell, or if Simon's problems reminded you of your own child's, then there's already quite a strong possibility that you too are affected in the same basic way.

All the people in the preceding pages, however different their personalities and their backgrounds and their individual stories, shared one common characteristic: they were all found to be food-allergic.

As you'll have noticed, they weren't affected by the same foods. Several reacted to wheat, some to dairy products, others instead (or as well) to such common foods as eggs, tomatoes, apples, oranges - even carrots.

Nor did they respond in the same way. Some, as you saw, put on weight. Others lost it. Others gained weight, lost it, gained again. Most, as well, faced other - different - problems, both mental and physical, besides their long-lasting battle to gain (or lose) weight.

Yet, hard to believe though it may seem, all their individual difficulties had the same underlying cause. **They - and thousands like them - are quite unable to cope with everyday foods which cause no trouble to others.**

This seems an extraordinary diagnosis. And what, at first sight, makes it even harder to accept is that it's the foods most frequently eaten that cause the most problems. These include not only things we already feel a bit guilty about (chocolate, sweets, cakes) but a whole range of all those we think of as 'good for us.'

Heading the list are such staples as:
    milk
    bread
    cereal
    cheese
    eggs
    oranges

potatoes

tomatoes

– and many others.

Because reactions are individual, the same food can cause opposite results in two different people; so that, like Jill and Jessica, one person grows overweight while another becomes underweight. Very often the weight problems are accompanied by other symptoms. Someone who's overweight, for example, may suffer from bloating, constipation, stomach cramps; someone else who's underweight, from indigestion, diarrhoea and vomiting.

Besides symptoms like these – which can be clearly connected with food and eating – people suffer from a whole range of others where the link is far less obvious. Sometimes, indeed, it's hard to believe there could be any connection.

Yet whenever weight problems are accompanied by any persistent or recurrent symptoms, whether physical or mental, for which no real diagnosis has been made, food allergy should always be considered – even if only to make sure that it's a suspect which can be safely eliminated.

Perhaps, like many people first exposed to this idea, you are at the moment intrigued – but sceptical.

Well, you're in good company. Scepticism is the normal first reaction. It is after all extremely difficult to accept the notion that you should be unable to eat perfectly everyday things that everyone around you seems to be enjoying.

But if you can, for a moment, suspend your disbelief, you can see just *why* conventional diets – of whatever variety – simply wouldn't work for Jill or Thomas or any of the others you've been reading about. And just why – if you're food-allergic too – they haven't worked, don't work, and won't work for you.

Or, at least, they'll never work permanently.

They may, by coincidence, work temporarily. If, say, you go on a week's semi-fast on fruit alone, and you happen to be allergic to the cheese you normally enjoy several times a week, and the milk you drink in pints, you'll certainly lose weight.

But as soon as you return to anything like your normal pattern of eating, your problems will return. Indeed, you're likely to find them worse than ever.

Ordinary diets fail food-sensitive people because they make no allowances for individual responses.

Wholemeal bread is excellent for most – but very damaging for some. To suggest, as some diets do, that it should be eaten every day (or even several times a day) is to condemn people like Jill or Thomas to a very unhappy state of affairs. A pint of milk a day, whether skimmed or not, will produce results in milk-allergic people quite opposite to those intended.

Of course not every failed dieter, not every bony individual longing to put on weight, suffers from unsuspected allergies.

But certainly a sizeable proportion do.

If you've lost weight (perhaps more than once) – only to put it on again . . .

If you stay ultra thin – no matter how hard you try to flesh out a little . . .

If counting calories and weighing portions depresses you – but never seems to work . . .

If you're not only the wrong weight and the wrong shape, but you're also less than well in other ways (you're depressed, or tired, or spotty, or you get indigestion or headaches or sleep badly) – in other words, you're less than 100% fit. . .

Then the chances are very high that the A-Diet could be right for you.

WHAT MAKES THE A-DIET DIFFERENT FROM ANY OTHER?

1. It establishes the right diet for YOU. Not for the rest of your family or your best friend or your workmate, but the right one for you personally.

2. It's concerned with the overall balance of what you eat and drink. There's no weighing or measuring or counting.

3. Once through the initial establishing stages, you won't be hungry or feel deprived. On the contrary: you'll feel healthier and more energetic than ever before.

4. It's not a 'miracle diet'. There's nothing weird and wonderful

about it. It works because it establishes a way of cutting out things that are harmful for you and substituting those that aren't.

5. Although in fact many allergic people do make dramatic weight losses (or gains) on establishing their proper diets, this isn't meant to be a crash diet. Your A-Diet is designed to be at least long-term – and quite possibly lifetime.

Though you may be able (if you wish) to modify it later, it's a diet which will keep you the right weight (for you), the right shape (for you), fit and healthy and (hopefully) happy right through life.

6. Because it's a truly individual diet, only you can work it out – just as only you can tell whether a pair of shoes fits you or not. This book explains, step by step, exactly how to go about it. (Though you don't necessarily need to read it all – more about this later.)

There's nothing complicated about it. All you need is an open mind, perseverance, and the determination to succeed.

QUESTIONS, QUESTIONS

By this time, queries are bound to have been popping into your mind. Here are some of those most frequently asked.

1. *If I really am food-allergic, surely I'd have noticed before for myself?*
Some people do in fact find out for themselves – sometimes as a result of changing their diet while on holiday or failing to eat during an illness.

But it's not at all easy to detect spontaneously. This sort of allergy is different from the kind you already know about: when certain individuals get blotches after eating strawberries, or are sick after eating shellfish. In fact, it's often known as 'masked' allergy, because it's so well concealed that it's hard to spot.

It acts in much the same way as alcohol. If you, like Jill, were affected by wheat, you'd feel fine as long as you got your regular fix of bread or biscuits. Yet at some point your body would rebel at having to cope what is, for it, a hostile substance. That's when your weight problems (and quite possibly a whole range of other symptoms) would start.

At the same time, you'd still go on getting a boost from the very food (or foods) doing you the most harm. So you can see how easy it is for people to go on for years without the slightest suspicion that food allergies could be involved.

2. *But even if it never occurred to me, surely – if it's really a possibility – some doctor would have mentioned it at some point?*

Unfortunately, the majority of GPs and specialists are still barely aware that food allergy exists, so they're very unlikely to consider it – even as part of a diagnosis.

3. *If food allergy could really cause problems like mine, however can it happen that most doctors know nothing about it?*

Doctors aren't trained to look for or recognise it.

Until very recently, little was taught about the role of nutrition in general, and even less about the existence of individual responses to foods.

'Allergy' is not a recognised medical specialisation (in the way that, for example, Rheumatology is). Therefore there are no specialists to teach, and a lack of students who can later go out to teach others.

It still takes a determined effort for doctors to find out about food allergy for themselves.

Although the first major book on this subject* was published as long ago as 1905, and although other important books and papers have been appearing for as long as sixty years, they never succeeded in attracting general medical attention.

In this country, it's only in the past few years that food allergy has begun to arouse any informed interest at all. 1976 saw the publication of Dr Richard Mackarness's *Not All In The Mind* (Pan); and two years later the first study devoted specifically to food allergy* was published in a leading medical journal.

Since then several further important research papers have been printed both here and abroad. However, since doctors are hard-pressed people – and the average GP is exposed to over 2 million words a year of drug details alone – it's not surprising that they find it impossible to keep up with the flood of medical information.

So, although interest is growing rapidly, the actual number of doctors aware of the significance of food allergy remains small. Statis-

The Food Factor In Disease, F.W.E. Hare, Longmans
*'Food allergy – fact or fiction?' *Lancet*, 25.2.1978

tically speaking, the odds are heavily against your having encountered one of them.

4. *But over the years I've seen a number of different doctors – both GPs and consultants. Surely I might have expected at least one of them to have suggested it – if that really is my basic problem?*

Surprisingly, the more doctors you've seen, the less probable it is that anyone would have thought of food allergy.

Patients who have a variety of symptoms (and this is a characteristic of many food-allergic people) find themselves referred to different specialists – perhaps at the same hospital, but in different clinics. There's rarely any inter-departmental consultation.

This means that if you saw, for example, a gastro-enterologist about your constant stomach pains, a dermatologist about your mystery rash, plus perhaps a psychologist about your headaches and depression, none of them is likely to have considered the whole picture you presented.

Although it's precisely this mixture of symptoms which points to the possibility of food allergy, the pattern won't reveal itself to specialists treating each one in isolation. It's therefore quite exceptional for the diagnosis of food allergy to be considered.

5. *Does all this mean then that food allergy is in fact rare?*

On the contrary. Even a very conservative estimate is that it affects at least one in 20. Some doctors would put it very much higher indeed: at one in 10, or even one in five.

6. *Could an NHS allergy clinic find out if I was food allergic?*

In the past, almost certainly not. Today, there are a few clinics scattered through the country which are interested in food allergies and will carry out investigations through diet changes; but at present these are still very thin on the ground.

Others have neither the interest nor the experience to analyse or advise.*

7. *Do all food-allergic people have weight problems?*

No. But overweight, underweight, and fluctuations of weight together make up one of the five most common symptoms of food allergy. (The A-Diet, incidentally, will also help those who suffer from other symptoms, quite apart from weight problems. See p. 121.)

*see also 'Allergy' opposite.

'Allergy'

One difficulty is that for many years now medical opinion has been tied up in debates about what actually constitutes 'allergy'.

For classical immunologists, allergy is a self-damaging immunological response brought about by antibodies or lymphocytes; and therefore detectable by certain blood tests.

According to this definition, where the mechanism is not known (and blood tests reveal no changes), there can be no true 'allergy'. Some specialists consider that in such a case neither allergy nor something that looks like it can exist at all.

Others accept that it may exist, but prefer not to term it 'allergy' but instead 'idiosyncracy' or 'hypersensitivity'.

Moreover, what appears to be an allergic response may in fact be due to any one of a number of causes.

Our language at present lacks precisely defined words which are both readily understood and generally acceptable to distinguish properly between different types of 'allergy'.

Therefore, throughout this book, 'allergy' is used to mean any type of altered reaction (abnormal response), whether the precise mechanism is known or not.

Nor, of course, are all those with weight problems food-sensitive. It's time to find out how likely it is that you're an (as yet) undiagnosed sufferer.

Now turn the page and fill in all the answers to the Top Twenty Questions. . . . .

CHAPTER 3

COULD YOU BE FOOD-ALLERGIC?

Doctors who are experienced in examining and treating patients for suspected food allergy don't pluck such a diagnosis out of thin air. They search for clues in the patient's past history and present way of living. Some of these were present in all the cases quoted on pages 7–12.

If you too are affected, there will be clues as well in your own life and background. This quiz is designed to pick them out.

1. Is there any particular food or drink (or perhaps even more than one) which you crave for and eat (or drink) as often as you can?

Yes   No

2. Is there any food or drink (or more than one) which you know from experience makes you feel ill in some way?

Yes   No

3. Does food play a very important part in your life?

Yes   No

4. Have you ever binged? (This means: have you ever eaten far more than you needed, and *not been able to stop?*)

Yes   No

5. Have you ever – apart from periods of actual illness – totally lost your appetite, and not wanted to eat at all?

Yes   No

6. Do you suffer, or have you ever suffered, from any illness (such as hayfever, asthma or eczema) which is known to be caused (or partly caused) by allergies?

Yes   No

7. Do you know from experience (or have tests shown) that you react to something you breathe in (such as dust mites, animal hairs, tree or grass pollen)?

Yes   No

8. Do you know from experience (or have tests shown) that you can react to something you touch – or which touches you (e.g. certain flowers, detergents, cosmetics)?

Yes   No

9. Were you bottle-fed from birth (if you know)?

Yes   No

10. Did you, as a child, have frequent attacks of colic, tonsillitis, earache or conjunctivitis?

Yes   No

11. Apart from your weight problems, do you have any physical symptoms *at all* which persist, or keep reappearing, for which neither your GP nor any specialist can find any real cause?

Yes   No

12. Do you have any emotional or mental problems which seem unnecessary or excessive – depression, or anxiety, or panic attacks, or a general woolly-headedness?

Yes   No

13. Would anybody else in your family (parents, grandparents, brothers, sisters, children, uncles, aunts, cousin) answer 'Yes' to any of the questions from 7–11 inclusive?

Yes   No

14. Do you regularly or frequently use any medically-prescribed or over-the-counter drugs?

Yes   No

15. Do you know that you react adversely to any medical drug or drugs?

Yes   No

16. *(Females only)* Do you use, or have you ever used, the contraceptive pill?

Yes   No

17. Are you frequently exposed to chemicals either at home or at work? (This could include, for example, living on a busy road or near agricultural land subject to chemical farming; actually handling chemicals as part of your work, or simply being in the presence of chemicals used by others.)

Yes   No

18. Do you smoke, or are you often in the presence of smokers?

Yes   No

19. Does your diet regularly include processed or packaged foods or takeaways?

Yes No

20. Do you frequently feel under considerable stress, either at home or at work?

Yes No

How many times did you tick 'Yes'?

The higher your score, the higher the odds that allergies do indeed play a part in your weight problem.

Even as few as three to five positive answers could be significant.

Here, very briefly, is a look at the quiz, question by question, to explain what 'yes' replies could indicate.

1. Food allergy often has an addictive element. As already explained on the page before, it can act in much the same way as alcohol. Individuals can become hooked on the food(s) that are actually doing them harm. If you're keenly attached to a particular food or drink, to the extent that you know you'd really miss it if deprived of it, then the chances are high that you're actually allergic to it.

2. If you've happened to discover that a food or drink positively disagrees with you, then you already know that you're capable of being food-sensitive. It's quite on the cards that you're also being affected by other foods you don't suspect.

3. It's not 'normal' for food to play a dominant role in most people's lives. (We're not talking here about a professional interest, as in the case of a writer of cookery books.) If you plan your life around your meals, or you don't dare to leave home unless you know you're carrying supplies with you, this indicates an abnormal reaction.

4. Bingeing may spring from complex roots, but the perversion of appetite is certainly, in a proportion of cases, related to food allergy: or to other dietary imbalances (see also *Zinc*, p. 211).

5. The same is true of a persistent or repeated lack of appetite.

6–8. The experience of doctors in this field shows that many food-allergic people also suffer from symptoms which are recognised as allergic in origin. If you already know that you're officially allergic to something – whether it's pollen or dust or cats or detergents – then the less surprising it would be to find you were also allergic to foods.

9. Breast-feeding is known to help to prevent the later development of allergies, as it protects the infant's immature immune system.

10. Typically, a food-allergic adult has a childhood background of

repeated or persistent minor illnesses.

11–12. Food-allergic people can also have any of a wide range of symptoms. These vary from the visibly physical (rashes, swollen joints), to the invisibly physical (stomach pains, back-aches), to the apparently psychological ('nerves', exhaustion). It is their persistence or recurrence, together with the absence of any real cause, that is the clue that their true origin could be allergy.

13. There's a strong family connection in allergy. Though it's possible to be the only one of your family to be affected, this is unusual. If any of your relatives show symptoms which you recognise as being at least possibly allergic in origin, then this again could be significant.

14. All drugs affect the way the body functions. If you use drugs other than occasionally, this could be contributing to the 'total overload' and thus help to bring about food allergy. (For more details, see p. 199.)

15. An adverse reaction to any medical drug (in its recommended dose) is an indication that your system does not respond in a typical way. The same individual susceptibility can lead to food allergy.

16. The contraceptive pill causes many changes in the body, the effects of which can last for some time after it's no longer taken. Among these is damage to the immune system (thus leading to the development of food allergies) and various mineral imbalances. (See p. 201.)

17. All exposure to chemicals adds to the total overload. Not only can it cause reactions to the individual chemicals, but it can also – by damaging the immune system – lead to the development of food allergies. (See p. 199.)

18. Smoking, like other chemicals, also damages the immune system, and therefore makes the development of food allergy more likely. Unfortunately, exposure to other people's smoking can also be harmful. (See p. 205.)

19. Certain packaged and processed foods contain chemical additives, which can both cause allergic reactions themselves and increase the chances of developing food allergies. (See p. 203.)

20. Stress doesn't in itself *cause* allergy. However, by putting pressure on the system, it makes the body less able to cope with the results of any substances (whether foods or chemicals) which are unsafe for it. If you've noticed that you tend to put on (lose) weight when you're under stress, it isn't necessarily the stress itself which is

24

the sole and direct cause – even though it may appear to be so. (See p. 101.)

By now you'll have a good idea of how well the diagnosis of food allergy might fit you; and in the next section you'll start right away on your preliminary detective work.

Allergy – More Details

You'll find further information about allergy as you continue through the book, and particularly in chapter 13. If, by the end, you want to know still more (and it is a fascinating subject), you'll find details of useful books in the Appendix. These all contain further reading lists, together with particulars of relevant scientific papers.

CHAPTER 4

AS YOU ARE NOW

Starting tomorrow, for the next eight days you're going to keep an unusual diary: an As You Are Now Diary. When you've finished, you'll have put together a lot of useful information – some of which will probably surprise you!

After that, you'll take a long look at it – with the help of the guidance on pages 51–8 – so that you end up with a good idea of whether or not you're indeed food-allergic. Your AYAN Diary will then be of invaluable help in planning your next step.

Turn to page 34 and look at the headings. You'll find some of them obvious; but others will probably puzzle you.

Here are some notes to fill you in on what to do.

DAY ONE

Enter the date when you start – tomorrow, unless there's a good reason why not! (You'll probably want to refer to this diary later, and it's useful to have confirmation of when you actually started.) Continue filling in dates each day.

WEIGHT AM PM

First thing tomorrow morning, weigh yourself after you've been to the loo and before you've had anything to drink.

At night, weigh yourself again immediately before you go to bed.

Repeat this every day.

FOODS/DRINKS

Every time during the day that you stop to have something to eat or drink, whether it's a meal or a snack, put a tick by every specific individual item you're eating/drinking in the long list on the left-hand side. (Apple [tick], cheese [tick], bacon [tick], and so on.) To do this, you think of what you're having as a collection of its various ingredients.

This means that often you'll have to stop and work out exactly what the ingredients are. If you're having fried fish fingers, for example, put ticks opposite fish, wheat (= breadcrumbs), salt and additives (if present). If you fry them in, say, groundnut oil, put a tick opposite 'nuts'; if in lard, put one against 'pork'.

Any items that don't fit in (there's not space for everything) add in the blanks at the base to think about later.

It's easy enough when it's 'carrots' or 'apples' or 'chicken', or you've cooked something yourself and know exactly what you've used. It's more complicated when it's something you've bought already prepared, or had cooked for you.

Ask questions and read labels.

Don't worry though if you can only get your analysis approximately right. That's all that matters at this point.

Quantities aren't that important at the moment. However, if you have at any one time what you would consider an extra large or double portion, put down two ticks instead of one.

The separate *meats* include all cuts, and any recipes incorporating these.

Thus, 'beef', 'veal', 'lamb' includes liver, kidneys, mince, sausages, pies, pâtés and so on.

'Pork' similarly includes any part or product (e.g. sausages, pates, pies, salami etc); with the exception of bacon and ham, which share a separate column.

'Chicken' and 'turkey' also include any foods with chicken or turkey as part of the ingredients: don't forget pies, pâtés and rissoles.

'Corn (maize)' includes everything derived from corn: e.g. sweetcorn, corn on the cob, cornflour, cornmeal, corn flakes, corn oil, and sweeteners made from corn (though it's not always possible to identify these).

'Wheat' includes everything derived from wheat: wheat cereals such as Weetabix and Shredded Wheat, bread, breadcrumbs, batter, flour, pastry, biscuits, cakes, bran (which is usually wheat), pasta etc.

'Yeast' is present in all bread (except specialist unleavened bread), certain cakes and pastries (e.g. croissants), yeast extracts (e.g. Marmite), and all alcoholic drinks.

For any foods made only partly from meat, you'll need to put ticks not only in the appropriate meat column, but also opposite the other various ingredients. For something like sausages, for example, you'd put a tick against 'pork' or 'beef'; plus probably a tick for wheat (most bought sausages contain 'rusk' which is usually wheat-based); plus – again probably – a tick in the additives column. And so on.

Similarly, if you have tea (or coffee) with milk and sugar, you put ticks against tea (or coffee) *and* milk *and* sugar. You put one tick per each cup.

If you eat any tinned, packaged or processed foods, read the labels and tick all the ingredients.

'Sugar' means a tick for every time this is included in any food: not just tea or coffee, as above, but e.g. in jam, marmalade, biscuits, cakes, tinned foods etc (read every label). For this purpose, 'sugar' includes 'caramel', 'dextrose', 'fructose', 'glucose', 'lactose', 'maltose', 'sucrose'.

'Additives* is here a term used as shorthand to include anything with an E-number, or 'artificial sweetener' or 'artificial flavouring' or 'preservative' or 'anti-oxidant' or 'colouring' or 'flavour enhancer' or monosodium glutamate (MSG).

At the end of each day, add up the ticks opposite each item, and fill in the number in the appropriate box.

ANY EXERCISE TAKEN

This includes any exercise, whether incidental or intentional: walking to work, jogging, cycling, loading crates, vacuuming, digging, swimming, squash etc.

*Some additives – eg certain colourings and anti-oxidants are of natural rather than synthetic origin; however, for the purposes of this diary they can for the time being be grouped together.

ANY SYMPTOMS

Put down here anything you notice about yourself and your health, whether it's absolutely specific ('spots on back') or somewhat vague ('slight ache in wrists'). Enter both when symptoms start and when they stop.

HOW YOU FEEL

This is the chance to note your moods. Jot down whether you feel exhilarated or depressed or irritable or whatever.

DRUGS

This includes any prescription or over-the-counter drugs: including the Pill. Write down any you take: the quantity and the frequency.

CHEMICALS YOU'RE IN CONTACT WITH

This means any chemicals you actually use, and any you're aware of in your surroundings: such as bleach, air fresheners, petrol fumes, hair sprays, paint, lavatory cleaners etc. A useful tip is to put down everything which smells but is not of natural origin.

HAPPENINGS

Note down here anything which doesn't take place every day: a visit, a fresh assignment, a quarrel, new equipment – anything which seems to you to be worth remarking.

Don't procrastinate. Start first thing tomorrow – unless for some reason (perhaps you're on holiday) your eating pattern is likely to be unusual.

Don't make any attempt to modify your diet in any way. If you normally have doughnuts for elevenses, don't let a feeling of lurking guilt push you into switching to raw carrots. You're not playing *Truth* for the sake of anyone else. You simply want to establish a clear picture, from a weight and health point of view, of you as you are now.

And now put the scales somewhere you'll see them first thing in the morning, so you don't have a chance to forget. . . .

For the Record

This is optional. If you think it might encourage you, fill it in. (If you do, it could be a good idea to read p. 54 at the same time.) If you'd rather not, and think it would depress you, leave it out.

Weight

Measurements

Chest	Upper arms
Neck	Upper thighs
Waist	Wrists
Hips	Ankles

How your skin looks

Your present state of health

How you feel

Any other comments

CHAPTER 5

YOUR AS YOU ARE NOW DIARY

DAY ONE

FOODS/DRINKS	WEIGHT	AM	PM

TOTAL EXERCISE TAKEN

ANY SYMPTOMS

ADDITIVES
APPLE
ALCOHOL
BACON OR HAM
BANANA
BEANS
BEEF OR VEAL
BUTTER
CABBAGE
CARROTS
CAULIFLOWER
CHEESE
CHICKEN
CHOCOLATE
COFFEE
CORN (MAIZE)
CUCUMBER
EGG

HOW YOU FEEL	DRUGS	CHEMICALS YOU'RE IN CONTACT WITH	HAPPENINGS

FISH
GRAPEFRUIT
LAMB
LEMON
LETTUCE
MILK
MUSHROOMS
NUTS
OATS
ONION
ORANGES
PEAS
PEPPERS
PORK
POTATO
RICE
SALT
SUGAR
TEA
TOMATO
TURKEY
TURNIP, SWEDE
WHEAT
YEAST
YOGURT
ANY OTHER ITEMS

DAY TWO

FOODS/DRINKS	WEIGHT AM	PM

TOTAL EXERCISE TAKEN

ANY SYMPTOMS

ADDITIVES
APPLE
ALCOHOL
BACON OR HAM
BANANA
BEANS
BEEF OR VEAL
BUTTER
CABBAGE
CARROTS
CAULIFLOWER
CHEESE
CHICKEN
CHOCOLATE
COFFEE
CORN (MAIZE)
CUCUMBER
EGG
FISH

HOW YOU FEEL

DRUGS

CHEMICALS YOU'RE
IN CONTACT WITH

HAPPENINGS

GRAPEFRUIT
LAMB
LEMON
LETTUCE
MILK
MUSHROOMS
NUTS
OATS
ONION
ORANGES
PEAS
PEPPERS
PORK
POTATO
RICE
SALT
SUGAR
TEA
TOMATO
TURKEY
TURNIP, SWEDE
WHEAT
YEAST
YOGURT
ANY OTHER ITEMS

37

DAY THREE

WEIGHT AM PM

FOODS/DRINKS

TOTAL EXERCISE TAKEN

ANY SYMPTOMS

ADDITIVES
APPLE
ALCOHOL
BACON OR HAM
BANANA
BEANS
BEEF OR VEAL
BUTTER
CABBAGE
CARROTS
CAULIFLOWER
CHEESE
CHICKEN
CHOCOLATE
COFFEE
CORN (MAIZE)
CUCUMBER
EGG
FISH

GRAPEFRUIT
LAMB
LEMON
LETTUCE
MILK
MUSHROOMS
NUTS
OATS
ONION
ORANGES
PEAS
PEPPERS
PORK
POTATO
RICE
SALT
SUGAR
TEA
TOMATO
TURKEY
TURNIP, SWEDE
WHEAT
YEAST
YOGURT
ANY OTHER ITEMS

HOW YOU FEEL

DRUGS

CHEMICALS YOU'RE IN CONTACT WITH

HAPPENINGS

39

DAY FOUR

FOODS/DRINKS	WEIGHT	AM	PM

TOTAL EXERCISE TAKEN

ANY SYMPTOMS

ADDITIVES
APPLE
ALCOHOL
BACON OR HAM
BANANA
BEANS
BEEF OR VEAL
BUTTER
CABBAGE
CARROTS
CAULIFLOWER
CHEESE
CHICKEN
CHOCOLATE
COFFEE
CORN (MAIZE)
CUCUMBER
EGG
FISH

HOW YOU FEEL

DRUGS

CHEMICALS YOU'RE
IN CONTACT WITH

HAPPENINGS

GRAPEFRUIT
LAMB
LEMON
LETTUCE
MILK
MUSHROOMS
NUTS
OATS
ONION
ORANGES
PEAS
PEPPERS
PORK
POTATO
RICE
SALT
SUGAR
TEA
TOMATO
TURKEY
TURNIP, SWEDE
WHEAT
YEAST
YOGURT
ANY OTHER ITEMS

DAY FIVE

FOODS/DRINKS	WEIGHT	AM	PM

TOTAL EXERCISE TAKEN

ANY SYMPTOMS

ADDITIVES
APPLE
ALCOHOL
BACON OR HAM
BANANA
BEANS
BEEF OR VEAL
BUTTER
CABBAGE
CARROTS
CAULIFLOWER
CHEESE
CHICKEN
CHOCOLATE
COFFEE
CORN (MAIZE)
CUCUMBER
EGG
FISH

HOW YOU FEEL

DRUGS

CHEMICALS YOU'RE IN CONTACT WITH

HAPPENINGS

GRAPEFRUIT
LAMB
LEMON
LETTUCE
MILK
MUSHROOMS
NUTS
OATS
ONION
ORANGES
PEAS
PEPPERS
PORK
POTATO
RICE
SALT
SUGAR
TEA
TOMATO
TURKEY
TURNIP, SWEDE
WHEAT
YEAST
YOGURT
ANY OTHER ITEMS

DAY SIX

FOODS/DRINKS	WEIGHT AM	PM

TOTAL EXERCISE TAKEN

ANY SYMPTOMS

ADDITIVES
APPLE
ALCOHOL
BACON OR HAM
BANANA
BEANS
BEEF OR VEAL
BUTTER
CABBAGE
CARROTS
CAULIFLOWER
CHEESE
CHICKEN
CHOCOLATE
COFFEE
CORN (MAIZE)
CUCUMBER
EGG
FISH

44

HOW YOU FEEL

DRUGS

CHEMICALS YOU'RE
IN CONTACT WITH

HAPPENINGS

GRAPEFRUIT
LAMB
LEMON
LETTUCE
MILK
MUSHROOMS
NUTS
OATS
ONION
ORANGES
PEAS
PEPPERS
PORK
POTATO
RICE
SALT
SUGAR
TEA
TOMATO
TURKEY
TURNIP, SWEDE
WHEAT
YEAST
YOGURT
ANY OTHER ITEMS

DAY SEVEN

FOODS/DRINKS	WEIGHT AM	PM

TOTAL EXERCISE TAKEN

ANY SYMPTOMS

ADDITIVES
APPLE
ALCOHOL
BACON OR HAM
BANANA
BEANS
BEEF OR VEAL
BUTTER
CABBAGE
CARROTS
CAULIFLOWER
CHEESE
CHICKEN
CHOCOLATE
COFFEE
CORN (MAIZE)
CUCUMBER
EGG
FISH

HOW YOU FEEL

DRUGS

CHEMICALS YOU'RE
IN CONTACT WITH

HAPPENINGS

GRAPEFRUIT
LAMB
LEMON
LETTUCE
MILK
MUSHROOMS
NUTS
OATS
ONION
ORANGES
PEAS
PEPPERS
PORK
POTATO
RICE
SALT
SUGAR
TEA
TOMATO
TURKEY
TURNIP, SWEDE
WHEAT
YEAST
YOGURT
ANY OTHER ITEMS

47

DAY EIGHT

FOODS/DRINKS	WEIGHT AM	PM

TOTAL EXERCISE TAKEN

ANY SYMPTOMS

ADDITIVES
APPLE
ALCOHOL
BACON OR HAM
BANANA
BEANS
BEEF OR VEAL
BUTTER
CABBAGE
CARROTS
CAULIFLOWER
CHEESE
CHICKEN
CHOCOLATE
COFFEE
CORN (MAIZE)
CUCUMBER
EGG
FISH

HOW YOU FEEL

DRUGS

CHEMICALS YOU'RE
IN CONTACT WITH

HAPPENINGS

GRAPEFRUIT
LAMB
LEMON
LETTUCE
MILK
MUSHROOMS
NUTS
OATS
ONION
ORANGES
PEAS
PEPPERS
PORK
POTATO
RICE
SALT
SUGAR
TEA
TOMATO
TURKEY
TURNIP, SWEDE
WHEAT
YEAST
YOGURT
ANY OTHER ITEMS

49

CHAPTER 6

EIGHT DAYS LATER

After eight days of individual detective work, you now have a record which is unique to you. No one else will have eaten or drunk exactly the same things at the same times, reacted in the same way, taken the same kinds of exercise or been exposed to the same chemicals.

So let's take a closer look.

FOODS/DRINKS

A. Write down here any individual items which received at least one tick on seven or eight days of the diary.

The foods and drinks you're most likely to be allergic to are those you eat or drink most regularly. *So you can be particularly suspicious of anything which appears above.*

B. Now note those which were ticked on four, five, or six days.

You should be wary too of any items appearing in this second list.

C. Now check those which were ticked on two or three days.

It's possible to be, or become, allergic to foods or drinks taken even as comparatively rarely as twice a week – provided that this continues regularly over a period. So, although these make up a less likely group, you should at this point *include them too as possibilities.*

D. Cross out, on the following list, any item which *doesn't* feature in your lists A, B, C above.

Put three stars against any which appears in list 1; two for any in list 2; 1 for any in list 3.

Then note down also the total number of ticks each has had during the 8 days.

Bacon + ham
Cheese
Chocolate
Corn
Eggs
Milk
Oranges
Potatoes
Sugar
Tomatoes
Wheat

As you'll have guessed, these items have been picked out because they're known to be among those most likely to cause problems. (The list is arranged alphabetically – not in any order of probability.)

Both the number of stars and the total of ticks are significant. You have to consider them together. You could, for example, have three stars and 32 ticks; or three stars but only eight ticks – or just one star and the same eight ticks.

On the whole, a high star rating *plus* a high number of ticks is a good indication that whatever-it-is is going to prove one of your problems. A high star rating, even with a lower number of ticks, is also likely to be significant. On the other hand, a lower star rating plus an unusually high number of ticks *could* indicate that you're capable of over-indulging when you get the chance.

Turn the answers to Questions 1–4 over in your mind. If you *are* allergic – and the answers below will go some way to confirm whether or not this is the case – then the chances are high that most (if not all) of your unsafe foods are noted above.

5. How many ticks did you get for sugar?

If you had more than a very modest number of sugar-ticks, then sugar is a problem for you, whether or not you are, strictly speaking, allergic to it. (For more details on sugar, see pages 182 and 183.)

All would-be dieters know that sugar is a baddy (but that certainly doesn't mean that they always resist temptation). And even those who always make a point of never taking it in tea or coffee often fail to realise how much is hidden in what they're eating or drinking.

You may have been surprised to find how often you've had to add a sugar-tick after reading the labels – even on savoury foods. In fact, over the country as a whole, 60% of sugar is eaten as part of processed or packaged foods.

Remember, when you read a label, that contents are listed in descending order. So if sugar appears as item number 2, then there's more sugar than anything else except for item number 1. If you haven't checked on this before, it will probably come as a shock to discover how often sugar comes high (often next to the top) in the lists of contents.

In some cereals, for example, sugar can amount to a fifth or even a quarter of the total. This means that whenever you pour, say, five tablespoons of cereal into your bowl you may be eating at least one tablespoon, and possibly more, of sugar.

As you may have discovered, sugar is also present in the most unlikely foods: baked beans, tinned soups, beefburgers, ketchup, ham. If, as well, you do add sugar to tea or coffee, you may also have been taken aback – many people are – to discover just how many sugar-ticks you've been jotting down.

You can see how quickly all those odd teaspoons could together add up to a whole bagful.

6. How many ticks for tea?
   How many for coffee?
   How many for tea plus coffee combined?

Are you mainly a tea-drinker? And do you have 40 ticks (or more) for tea?

Or are you a coffee-drinker, with 40 ticks (or more) for coffee?

Or, if you drink both, is your combined total 40 or over?

In any of these cases, you're drinking more of either (or both) than many doctors would consider wise.

It's not that the tea or coffee will *directly* affect your weight (although if you take sugar with it it certainly may); but either can affect the way your body functions, so that you're more likely to develop allergies to other foods.

(And you can, of course, easily become allergic to the tea or coffee itself. For more about this, see p. 75 and 135.)

WEIGHT

Did your weight remain more or less stable throughout the week?

If not, did it rise (or fall) more than 1 lb on one or more occasions?

If so, look at the preceding 24 hours.

Was there a specific food (or drink) you'd eaten or drunk in unusually large quantities?

Or had you, on the contrary, during this period *not* eaten or drunk something you normally eat or drink? (Perhaps you ran out of bread, or the milk turned sour?)

Or did you eat an unusual variety of a food or drink (a different cheese, perhaps)?

If you spotted anything unusual along these lines, write the items concerned down here.

(*Note for women* If a weight change during this time appears to be connected with a period, this may be only an *indirect* rather than a *direct* consequence of hormonal changes; that is, the extra stress on your system may have added to your 'total overload,'* and thus caused you to react more strongly to foods which at other times you are better able to tolerate. It is therefore still important that you take note of what you have eaten or drunk during this time.)

If you can see nothing different in any 24 hours before a marked rise (or drop) in weight, then look as far back as the preceding 48 hours: i.e. two full days before you noted the change of weight.

Were there any similar alterations in your normal diet at any point during this time? In particular, look out for any changes in whatever grain-based foods you normally eat. (These include bread, cereals, pasta and so on.) Such foods can bring about reactions delayed for two or even three days after being taken.

Note here anything you have reason to suspect.

*see p. 206.

ANY SYMPTOMS

Note down here any symptoms which you had. If any occurred on more than one day, add the number of days down after the symptom.

Were there any reasons that you know of for any of these symptoms? (You'd eaten food which you suspected wasn't fresh; or you'd had upsetting news immediately before a meal.) In this case, ignore the symptoms for the time being – the chances are they're not relevant.

But if, on the other hand, there seems to be no obvious reason that you can pin down for your symptom(s), then this could certainly be significant. It suggests that reactions to foods (or chemicals) *could* be involved.

Again – as with your check on weight fluctuations – note down beside each symptom:

any food or drink eaten in unusual quantities within the preceding 24 hours;

any food or drink you'd unusually gone without within the preceding 24 hours;

any unusual kind of food or drink you'd had within the preceding 24 hours;

any food or drink you'd eaten conspicuously more *or* less of (or eaten an unusual kind of) within the preceding 48 hours.

Symptoms: Possibly involved foods or drinks.

DO ANY SYMPTOMS AND WEIGHT CHANGES COINCIDE?

If so, note them down here.

In this case, of course, any suspect foods and drinks will also coincide.

Note these down here.

Do any of the foods or drinks you've just written down appear in any of Lists A–D at the beginning of the chapter (p. 51)?

If so, put the individual foods or drinks down opposite the appropriate list.

List A:

List B:

List C:

List D:

Any foods or drinks now appearing above in both lists A and D are very suspect indeed; suspect if in list B; and still suspect (though less so) if appearing in list C.

However, even if you haven't been able so far to observe any weight changes, or to note any symptoms; or – if you have – have failed to find any direct associations between these and your diet; it's still possible that foods and drinks may be involved.

It's very often possible to spot a connection even after as short a time as eight days, but it can take longer to detect the first clues. And it certainly takes longer to prove the case. That's what the next chapters are about.

ANY EXERCISE

On how many days did you take some form of exercise?

If your chart shows this happened on less than six of the eight days, then you're not giving your body a chance. Ideally, you should rate 8 out of 8. Anything less than 4 is very revealing.

Physical activity helps your body to function correctly. Although it's true that we're all individuals born with different metabolic rates, that doesn't mean that they're immutably fixed forever. We doubtless all know at least one thin, lively child who turned into an overweight, lethargic teenager.

It's perfectly possible to step up your metabolic rate, and this is desirable whether or not you turn out to be allergic. (For more about this, see p. 98.)

HOW YOU FELT

Were you reasonably even-tempered during this period? Or did you notice marked changes of emotion? Were these caused by actual events? And do you think – looking back – that how you felt was a justified and reasonable response? If so, then for present purposes you can discount your reactions.

If however they now seem to you excessive, or if on reflection you can't see why you behaved that way at all, then any changes of mood could be significant.

If the days on which you noticed such feelings corresponded with days on which you observed *either* changes of weight *or* symptoms, or both, then this helps to confirm the probability that you're food-allergic.

Even if you've so far discovered no such obvious link, bear the possibility in mind. It could still exist.

DRUGS

You may perhaps be one of those who end up disconcerted to realise just how many medicines they habitually take.

Does your list prominently feature common over-the-counter remedies? Although these are less powerful than prescribed drugs, they may still cause allergic reactions in themselves; and, when taken regularly, contribute to the possibility of food allergy. (Incidentally, you may like to be reassured that most people who successfully sort out their food allergy problems find they no longer have any call for their indigestion tablets, laxatives, pain-killers etc.)

If you're taking drugs prescribed by your GP, these also, of course, add to the chemical load.

Whatever the source of those you're taking, if they play an important part in your diary, please turn first to p. 199 *before* you go on to the next chapter.

If you're on the Pill, this also – as already mentioned on p. 24 – could have a direct bearing on the development of food allergy. Please turn to the short piece on page 201.

CHEMICALS

If you have more than the odd item jotted in this column, then everyday chemicals could play a vitally important part. (You'll perhaps have noticed how often in Chapter 1 various chemicals were mentioned as contributory causes.) Please read next the section on p. 198.

HAPPENINGS

You may be able to detect, from the notes in this column, some links that you never before suspected between places you visited, people you met, events that happened to you, and your overall health and well-being – and of course your weight. Even if any connection is only hazy at the moment, you may later find one that gradually takes shape.

This investigation is the essential key to your A-Diet.

As, bit by bit, you'll find out from now on.

CHAPTER 7

WHICH WAY FORWARD?

You've done a lot of the essential spade work.

What happens next depends on what you've discovered, how quickly you want to go, and how much of a gamble you're prepared to take.

You don't necessarily have to read the book right through from beginning to end. According to the different clues you already have, there are different routes you can choose to follow.

But before deciding which one to pick, look ahead at Chapters 8 and 10. Together, they form the core of the book.

YOUR ESSENTIAL DIET is the basis for your own A-Diet. If necessary, you'll continue to subtract and add to it until you discover the version which is right for you; but it will remain the permanent heart of your diet.

It's based on:

fresh foods of all kinds (apart from the restrictions mentioned below)

a very varied menu, with the avoidance of repetition

minimum use (at this stage) of milk

restricted use of grain-based foods

minimum use – or complete elimination, depending on the discoveries of your AYAN Diet – of common allergens, such as cheese, eggs, oranges

cutting out all processed and packaged foods

cutting out all or virtually all sugar.

YOUR ESSENTIAL LIVING PLAN is equally important. You should be prepared to consider this, too, as a permanent feature, and not just a passing stage.

How you live has an enormous effect on your health and weight problems in general, and on the development and treatment of food allergies in particular.

It's divided into two sections. The first looks at physical, and the second at mental factors which can affect your present and future progress.

Both chapters take up no more than 18 pages.

So read them, think about them, and then pick up again here.

Inevitably, in a book about weight problems and diet, there's a lot of emphasis on weight and weighing yourself. At the same time, I hope by the end you'll hardly feel the need to weigh yourself again.

Keeping a check on your weight is a useful guide to help you as you work out your diet. It's *changes* which are significant – not the weight in itself.

The A-diet is designed to help you reach the right weight for you. That, plus the Essential Living Plan, will also help you be the right shape for you. The idea of an imaginary 'target' weight has very little meaning.

People vary so enormously that two of the same sex and height can both be physically fit (and physically attractive), but with many pounds' weight difference between them.

Bulldogs Can't Make Greyhounds

Now is the time to choose your way ahead.

If the Essential Diet is very different from your present diet, and from any diet you've tried in the past, then you're strongly recommended to start by following this. Although not at all a difficult diet, it can mean a new way of looking at food, and involve different patterns of shopping, preparing and cooking meals. To begin with, it's enough to cope with any such changes, without committing yourself to any more drastic adaptations. However, bear in mind – as you follow it – any suspicions you now have as a result of your AYAN diet. Keep an eye open for any further reactions to any of your now suspect foods.

It's also possible for two to be the same height and the same weight – but one will look unhealthy, overweight and flabby, while the other will look fit and shapely.

A few people end up on their A-diet much the same weight as when they started, but very much healthier and a different shape. Their previous fat has changed to muscle. 'Cellulite' disappears.

At the same time, no amount of re-shaping is going to turn anyone into someone they were never designed to be. People come quite naturally in all shapes and sizes. We all have different genetic backgrounds and are born with bone structures of different proportions.

No amount of dieting will turn a bulldog into a greyhound – or vice versa. But the A-diet can turn you into a healthy, handsome bulldog (or greyhound); and ensure that you keep that way.

Back to Chapter 7

If the Essential Diet is fairly close to your present eating pattern, or you have in the past followed a similar diet for any length of time, then you may be keen to take further (different) steps as soon as possible.

But please note that this diet, although it naturally shares some of the characteristics of other healthy diets, is not the same. Don't underestimate how stressful you may find it to have to cut down heavily on both dairy products and grains – not to mention the other common allergens.

You could well find it worth while spending an extra eight – or even 16 days or more – following the Essential Diet before you introduce any variations.

However, if the Essential Diet is very close indeed to your present diet, and you have by now had very positive indications about the foods (drinks) causing your problems, then by all means move directly to Chapter 14.

Note that if you're contemplating losing (or gaining) more than a few pounds, you should always start by checking with your GP that there are no diagnosable medical causes for your over (under) weight.

Safe for Children and Teenagers as Well

Although, for convenience, 'you' is used throughout this book, this doesn't mean that the A-Diet is only suitable for adults. It's equally valid for any child or teenager with weight problems, whose answers to the page 21 Quiz indicate that allergies could be involved.

You may use the Essential Diet for them with every confidence. You may be concerned about the restrictions on milk. If so, please look now at the advice on pp. 139 and 154. Try to get the advice of a dietitian: you may be able to contact one through your GP.

However, do remember that a dietitian may still be unaware of the role of allergy. It's not unknown, for example, for parents to be recommended to continue giving their young child milk 'for the calcium', despite indications that this is a major cause of that individual child's problems.

It may be advisable for you, even at this stage, to look for further help. Turn to p. 132 for suggestions as to where to find it.

Possible Problems

1. Even with only the modest restrictions of the Essential Diet, your child (or teenager) could suffer from severe withdrawal symptoms (see p. 127). This depends largely on his/her previous diet. If major changes are involved, you may perhaps prefer to proceed slowly, and undertake the Essential Diet only in stages. You could, for example, start by cutting out for eight days foods and drinks containing additives. Next, you could eliminate sugar and anything containing sugar. After this, add the further restrictions on grains, following this by cutting down also on milk.

Only you, with your special knowledge of both your child's past diet and his/her temperament, can decide on how slowly or how fast to proceed.

2. Your child (or teenager) may become extremely awkward to live with. Although, once the initial stages are over, most children and teenagers both feel and look so much better that they're happy to keep to their diet because they want to, they're likely to start by fighting the changes being made – particularly since these may make them feel genuinely ill. The help given by a Support Group is especially welcome at this stage. Meanwhile, remind yourself that a) the more of a pain in the neck your son or daughter becomes, the more probable it is that you're on the right track; and b) it won't last for long.

3. Purely practical problems are almost the most difficult to overcome. You can feed your child or teenager the right diet at home, but what happens once they're outside your four walls? The biggest landmine for most parents is school milk and school dinners – and particularly school dinners.

Success in negotiating the hazards depends primarily on the individual policies of your local authorities. In many parts of the country it's currently impossible for a child to find a mid-day meal which corresponds at all to the Essential Diet. In certain others, where efforts are still being made to provide e.g. fresh food and salads, it should be possible to pick sufficient permitted foods.

Explaining the problem to both the class teacher and the head is important; but even with their co-operation it may be preferable to bring your child home every mid-day. If this is impossible – as it frequently is – then the only alternative is to prepare a suitable packed lunch.

This of course again has its dangers, as it's easy for children to be tempted by their friends' forbidden 'goodies'. However, experience shows that as time goes by they become less and less likely to succumb, as they begin to see clearly cause and unwanted effect.

They may not thank you now – but they will in the future.

CHAPTER 8

YOUR ESSENTIAL DIET

You'll see right away that your Essential Diet is both straightforward and tasty. There's nothing outlandish about it. It's suitable for anyone sharing the same meals – not just the would-be dieter – so it makes both planning and cooking simple.

Many ordinary diets slow you down. You eat so little that you find yourself with hardly any energy, and you end up doing the bare minimum. Your metabolism may slow right down in sympathy – so it's even possible to find yourself after days or weeks of struggle worse off than when you started.

This diet doesn't work like that. You can eat what you like of the long list of allowed foods. There's no need to go hungry. Far from feeling lethargic, the chances are that you'll find yourself with more energy than ever before.

Let's concentrate first on what you can eat – not on what you can't.

MEAT

You may eat any meat of any kind and any cut.

If you can buy fresh organically produced meat, so much the better: but otherwise any fresh or frozen meat, provided it has not been further processed in any way. Mince is all right, but beefburgers are not (unless they're guaranteed free of fillers and additives). Buy sausages only if you know they're 100% meat without cereal or additives (herbs are OK).

Aim to eat meat on not more than four or five days during the eight days of the diary. Don't eat meat from the same kind of animal on two successive days.

Quantities depend on your size, your work, and your leisure-time physical activity: anything from 4–10 oz of lean meat per portion; less of waste-free meats such as kidney and liver.

If 'ham' or 'bacon', appeared in your lists A or B on p. 51, then leave it/them out during this period. Otherwise, you may have either ham (or bacon) twice – or ham once + bacon once – with four days between the two occasions. (So after ham on Monday, no more ham – or bacon – until Friday).

Why this Diet?

This diet is based:
On the experiments, research and conclusions of (among others) Sir Robert McCarrison and Surgeon- Captain T.L. Cleave; and on adaptations of elimination and rotation diets developed and used by specialist doctors both here and in the United States.

1. In the first part of this century Sir Robert McCarrison carried out a series of experiments over many years which demonstrated that good health, both physical and mental, corresponded directly with the quality and correct balance of foods.

Specifically, he showed that a diet of unrefined grains, ample fresh fruits and vegetables, some dairy products and a little meat, was essential to the development of fit and healthy individuals, who would be neither too fat nor too thin, and who would grow into stable and sociable beings.*

Shortly afterwards, Cleave went on to demonstrate that not only obesity but a whole range of illnesses were due to what he called The Saccharine Disease: the consumption of refined carbohydrates, and in particular of white flour and sugar.*

He showed that these were damaging in three ways:

their consumption leads to a loss of fibre in the diet;

damage is caused to the system by the introduction of highly-concentrated elements;

over-eating such foods leads directly to the under-eating of other foods, particularly those containing essential proteins and vitamins.

2. McCarrison and Cleave demonstrated the importance of a good *general* diet.

However, it's been known for many years that certain foods which are otherwise nutritionally desirable can nonetheless be harmful for

*See Appendix

certain sensitive individuals.

Clinical ecologists (doctors experienced in the diagnosis and treatment of food and chemical allergies) have long observed that the more often a food or drink is consumed, the more likely it is that a sensitive individual will be allergic to it. (See also p. 119.)

In many cases it's necessary to identify and remove these items completely; and this is tackled in the elimination diets in Chapters 16–18.

Some people, though, can tolerate foods or drinks to which they are only slightly allergic as long as they consume them not more than once in every four days. (Such a diet is known as a 'rotation diet'.)

That's why, at this stage, the Essential Diet imposes the not-more-than-once-every-four-days rule on foods which are known to be major sources of trouble, such as bread, eggs, cheese etc.

FISH

You may eat any fish of any kind. Really fresh fish (which has not been previously frozen) is preferable. If you can't buy this then any kind of frozen fish will do, provided it's simply *fish* (fillets, steaks or whole fish). Don't buy any fish in batter, breadcrumbs or sauce; and no fish-cakes or pastes. You may buy tinned fish, as long as it's packed only in oil or brine with nothing else added. For the time being, steer clear of smoked fish.

Again, aim for variety. Don't eat the same type of fish over and over again.

As with meat, quantity again is variable, depending partly on your personal requirements, and partly on the compactness and boniness of the fish: from 4 oz to 12 oz.

POULTRY AND GAME

You may eat any of these: fresh is again preferable to frozen. Buy nothing in breadcrumbs or sauces or processed in any way.

Wild rabbit – if you can get it – is preferable to farmed, though farmed will do. Any kind of game you can find or afford is fine. Country-dwellers come off best here, but some major chains sell quite a variety in season. Venison is also now obtainable through some ordinary butchers.

Don't eat any one kind of poultry or game repetitively either, though if you have chicken one day, it's all right to switch to turkey or duck the next. (In some supermarkets now you can buy duck as well as turkey portions.)

VEGETABLES

If your diary shows that in the past you have – like the majority of people of this country – eaten vegetables comparatively rarely, then this is likely to amount to the biggest change for you. Vegetables are not going to be only a small garnish, but a large and important (and delicious) part of what you eat.

Eat as many vegetables as you like, as much of them as you like, and vary them as often as you can. Fresh vegetables in season are best. If you have problems with availability (as you may in some parts of the country and at certain times of year), then you may also eat frozen or (at a pinch) tinned vegetables. The frozen vegetables must be just vegetables: again, not in breadcrumbs, batter or sauce. Be sure to check the labels on tinned vegetables: salt is permitted, but nothing else – no sugar or any additives.

Right through the year, and wherever you are, you can sprout and eat a whole range of beans, pulses and grains (see p. 92).

Aim to eat every day at least one *raw vegetable* as salad.

Don't over-rely on any one kind of vegetable. Be particularly wary of potatoes and tomatoes. If either of these appeared on List A (p. 51), don't eat them at all during the first eight days. If they appeared on List B, don't eat either on more than two occasions during this period, and then only with a four-day interval between.

(If you're worried about what to do without potatoes, turn to p. 184.)

FRUIT

Eat some kind of fruit every day; and eat as much as you like, with the exception of citrus fruits. If any appeared on your List A, cut whichever-it-is out altogether; if on List B or C, cut your consumption down to twice a week.

Fresh fruit in season is ideal, but dried fruit is also useful, particularly in winter. You may also eat frozen or tinned fruit, provided it contains *no added sugar*. Again, variety is important.

NB If you're fortunate enough to be able to obtain – and afford – organically-grown vegetables or fruit (or even to grow your own), then these are a wise choice.

Fibre

Incidentally, fibre isn't simply a tablespoon of bran added to everything. This diet, with its emphasis on plenty of fruit and vegetables, both cooked and raw, is automatically high in fibre.

BREAD, CEREALS AND OTHER GRAINS

You may eat wholemeal bread, crisp-breads, oatcakes (without added sugar), any breakfast cereal which is simply grains with nothing added, wholemeal pasta, couscous, cornmeal (polenta), chapattis, rice (preferably brown), oats, barley, millet, rye: i.e. any grain in any form; but *only* as long as you follow this next very important rule.

You may not eat any one grain (or product from that grain) more frequently than on one day in any four days.

This means that if you eat, say, bread (or anything else made from wheat) on Monday, you mustn't eat wheat (or anything made from wheat) again until Friday. So if Monday is a wholemeal bread and wheat cereal-for-breakfast day, then you must not eat bread or wheat cereal for breakfast (or e.g. pizzas or spaghetti) until Friday.

The same rule applies for any other of the grains mentioned above.

FATS AND OILS

You may eat any butter or margarine; olive oil, sunflower oil or safflower oil.

At this stage, doctors with experience of food allergies in fact prefer butter, as it's been less processed and doesn't contain the mixture of ingredients that go into margarines. (It's true that a proportion of people on this diet will be found to be allergic to butter, but this is dealt with subsequently.) The selected oils are those less likely to cause reactions.

Saturated/Polyunsaturated Fats

You'll notice that this diet at this point treats the saturated/polyunsaturated argument as a side-issue; and considers primarily the proportion of fat + oil in the total diet.

Sixty per cent of the fat eaten in the average British diet is 'hidden' in processed foods. Since this diet allows no processed foods, the likelihood is that the total fat content will be drastically reduced. Oil is substituted for animal fats. Cheese and milk are either cut right down or eliminated altogether. Moreover, because of the restrictions on bread and other grain foods, many on this diet in any case eat less butter (or margarine) because they no longer have their daily sandwiches.

CHEESE

If cheese appears in List A or List B, then you must cut cheese out entirely. If it appears in List C, then you may eat it, but not more than twice during this period, and with four days between each occasion. (Eat only a modest helping – certainly not more than 3–4 oz.)

MILK

You may use a little milk for tea or coffee (see below) or to add to cereal; but you mustn't drink it or use it in cooking.

EGGS

If eggs appear on your Lists A or B, then leave them out altogether. Otherwise, you may eat eggs, but on not more than two occasions during this period (again, with four days between).

Warning

Some individuals who are highly allergic to any of the items which are either totally forbidden (e.g. chocolate, squash) or allowed only at four-day intervals (bread, cheese etc) may, even at this stage, suffer from withdrawal symptoms. (For more on this, see further on, p. 127.)

If, during these eight days, you feel tired, headachey, flu-ey, this may well be the cause. Despite what's said later in Chapter 11, if you do feel exhausted, for the time being forget about exercise. Rest as much as you can. Remember that the eight days will soon be over, and that by marking your symptoms (see pp. 121–3), and by working out what has caused them, you'll be on the way to solving your problems.

If, on eating for the second time a food which has become suspect, you experience a marked worsening of any symptoms, you may take either of the following.

2 tsp of sodium bicarbonate in ½ pint of water.

1 gm of soluble vitamin C, also in a large glass of water.

Don't take either more than twice in any one day.

NUTS

If any one kind of nut (peanuts, almonds) appeared in Lists A or B, then cut these out entirely. Otherwise, you may eat any kind of nuts, provided they're fresh and not salted. Again, don't eat any one kind repetitively.

SUGAR

As a concession, you may add a very little sugar – not more than one flat teaspoon – to tea or coffee (see below). You may also add a little (again, a very little) to breakfast cereal. If you feel you need to sweeten sharp cooked fruit – rarely necessary – add a little honey instead.

YOGURT

If yogurt appears on Lists 1 or 2, then cut it out altogether. Otherwise, you may use plain, unsweetened yogurt.

Vegetarians

Doctors confirm that, as a general rule, fewer vegetarians have weight problems (and indeed health problems) than non-vegetarians: vegetarians have made a deliberate decision to examine what they eat, and as a result cut out many potentially harmful substances.

However, because the range of foods that they eat is necessarily more limited, it's particularly important that they plan to eat a very varied diet. Their diet needs to be truly *vegetarian* – i.e. using plenty of vegetables and fruit – rather than simply non-carniverous.

Some vegetarians instead rely heavily on grains and cheese. When this happens, it's quite possible for them to become allergic to either or both.

If you're a vegetarian, your AYAN diary should indicate to you whether or not this could have happened in your case. Look particularly at your Lists A and B; and – in List D – at the number of ticks opposite wheat, milk, eggs and cheese. Check in particular how any weight fluctuations or changes of symptoms that you noticed could have corresponded with these major allergens.

Though difficult, it's not impossible to keep to the Essential Diet while excluding meat; certainly easier if you allow yourself fish. Be careful to observe the restrictions on grains and dairy products; for useful hints on alternatives, see pp. 154 and 160. Instead, use as wide a variety of vegetables, pulses and fruits as you can.

You can see that this 'diet' includes a very wide range of foods that you can eat – and enjoy.

In comparison, as you can see below, there's very little that is positively forbidden.

SUGAR

Apart from the very small allowance in tea or coffee or on cereal, sugar is completely ruled out. This means, of course, that you may not have *biscuits, cakes, sweets, chocolate, puddings etc.*

ARTIFICIAL SWEETENERS

You are advised against using these instead. Each of them is known to cause adverse reactions in certain individuals; and any one of them *may* affect the way your body functions.

SOFT DRINKS

You may not drink soft drinks at all: this includes all squashes and tinned or bottled beverages. (You may of course drink bottled natural mineral waters such as Malvern, Evian and Perrier.) Almost all such drinks contain added sugar and sweeteners; often additives and colourings; and some are caffein-related.

PURE FRUIT JUICES

Drink no pure fruit juices. Drinking them encourages over-consumption of the fruit concerned – it's easy, without realising it, to get through five or six oranges at a time in the form of juice. Instead, eat the whole fruit – at appropriate intervals where indicated. This also gives the body added fibre.

(You'll probably be able to reintroduce these later: see p. 130.)

PROCESSED OR PACKAGED FOODS

You may not for the moment eat any processed or packaged foods, with the exception of those mentioned above. Many such foods 1) contain hidden sugar and/or fat; 2) contain a variety of ingredients, to any one of which (e.g. wheat flour and dried milk) you may be allergic; 3) contain additives, which may a) be causing a number of symptoms without your guessing the connection, and b) be affecting the way your body reacts to other foods (see p. 204). (You'll be able to modify this later: see p. 130.)

TEA AND COFFEE

If your AYAN diary (check back to p. 34) shows that you've been drinking as much as five cups of tea or coffee, or five cups of tea-and-coffee combined, or even more, then strictly speaking you would do well to cut the tea or coffee (or tea and coffee) out altogether from this point. (For more on this, see p. 135.)

However, since the mere suggestion of this would be enough to turn a number of you off the thought of even starting on your Essential Diet, and since it's better to follow the diet while drinking a small amount of tea and coffee, rather than *not* follow it and continue drinking large amounts, here is a compromise.

You may drink up to three cups of any combination of tea or coffee; but no more. You are also advised to drink real (ground) and not instant coffee. As mentioned above, you may add a little milk and/or a little sugar.

If either the thought or the reality of this proves hard or impossible to face, then turn to p. 135 right away.

ALCOHOL

Again, if your diary shows that you've been drinking alcohol regularly every day, particularly if you take that alcohol consistently in the same form (you always drink beer, or always drink cider) then you should not drink alcohol at all during this 8-day period. However, if you do find the thought of total abstinence on top of a new diet too much to contemplate, then, at this stage, once more go for a compromise.

You may drink one glass of wine or half a pint of beer or cider once or twice a day: preferably with meals.

If you know you're going to have real problems sticking to this, then turn now to p. 135.

When you follow your Essential Diet, **your body receives a good balance of everything necessary for your health –**

including trace elements, vitamins and minerals.

While there's no need for hard and fast rules as to when you eat, or how often, for most people it makes sense to have three meals a day at fairly regular times. Make sure to eat a good breakfast.

You should be hungry before you start a meal – and you will, if you lead a reasonably active life – but it's unwise to let yourself get ravenous: that's the way to succumb to temptation and eat anything that's handy. Never go on eating from pure habit. When you stop feeling hungry, and start feeling full: stop.

Don't nibble. Don't eat things in passing. Don't gobble. Try to allow yourself a sensible amount of time for a meal. Sit down. Relax. Eat calmly.

If you only have a short time, eat a small meal. Allow yourself to enjoy what you're eating. If you're in company, join in the conversation. If you're on your own, perhaps listen to a favourite tape or programme.

How Much Should You Eat?

You'll have noticed that above there are hardly any guidelines as to quantities. This is because people's requirements vary so much that a fixed quantity is of little use. A tall, large individual doing hard physical work eight or ten hours a day needs far more fuel than someone else who is small and slightly built, works from a desk, and whose only exercise is to walk to the car and back. (Which is why you should consider Chapter 11 at the same time as this one.)

The more energy you expend, the more fuel you need. If you're in doubt, start with smaller quantities. Then, if you find you're left feeling hungry, add a little more.

You do need to be flexible about what you eat when. Perhaps this particularly applies to breakfast.

Breakfast doesn't *have to* be cereals, milk and sugar.

The Scots eat (or used to eat) herrings in oatmeal. It's perfectly possible to breakfast on fish, or chick peas, or lentils, or kidneys, or fish roe, or stewed apricots – or whatever you want that fits into the above diet. (If the thought of actual *food* for breakfast really upsets you, how about trying a short first-thing-in-the-morning walk to stir up your appetite?)

Until you succeed in working out your own new eating pattern, the main aim is to remain open-minded as to what you eat and when you eat it.

How am I going to manage?
Isn't it going to be very expensive?
Won't it mean a lot of extra work?
All these questions, and more, you'll find answered in Chapter 9.

CHAPTER 9

HELP AT HAND

Doctors who propose to their patients that they follow this diet – or something close to it – find that most of them react with a string of questions.

So here, briefly, are anwers to the three most often asked.

WON'T THIS DIET COST MUCH MORE?

It does depend, naturally, on how you've shopped and cooked before. But it certainly needn't be – and in practice it's possible for it to work out less.

If in the past you've spent money on soft drinks, biscuits, cakes, or any of the other items that you no longer need, then you save all that money right away.

Fresh vegetables and fruit in season are almost always less expensive than in any prepared form. Eaten raw in salads, or only lightly cooked, they're filling and go a long way.

Wholemeal grains and flour are more satisfying than refined, and so work out cheaper. Home-cooked pulses (beans, peas, lentils) cost much less than their prepared equivalents. If you want to be really enterprising, and sprout your own beans and make your own tofu (not difficult – instructions later), you can produce excellent contributions to meals for only a few pence.

Cheaper fish (coley, herring, mackerel) is just as tasty and nutritious as expensive. Tinned sardines and tinned mackerel are also good buys.

Some meat is certainly very expensive, but not all. Cheaper cuts may still be dearer than, say, sausages, but remember you're paying for meat alone – not for meat plus bread. Kidneys and liver, properly cooked, are considered delicacies in other countries, and work out at a really low cost per portion.

Of course most game (suggested as a possibility to add variety to the diet) is expensive; but pigeons are relatively cheap, and rabbit and poultry are always good value.

In fact, you can see that you might end up surprised by the economic results of your Essential Diet.

BUT WON'T IT MEAN A LOT MORE WORK?

It may take longer to shop – though not necessarily. What you buy will probably weigh more; so it's worth investing in a good trolley. There's one which splits into two for loading into a car which can be particularly useful.*

It tends to take longer to prepare meals from scratch than to open packets, but nonetheless there are plenty which are quick and easy to prepare: such as fish, soup, salad or stir-fried dishes.

It depends also how many others you're cooking for. If it's just for yourself, it really doesn't take long to chop up vegetables etc. for one. If you're cooking for a number, then co-opt help. If you can afford it, a food processor is particularly helpful in preparing quantities of vegetables for salads, pureeing for soup, etc.

Some meals take time in the cooking, rather than in the preparation, such as pulses and stews. Pressure-cookers and slow-cookers can both help here.

If you've not really cooked before, then everything will seem to take a long time to start with. But don't worry – you really will speed up with practice.

BUT SURELY COOKING IS A SKILL? HOW DO I KNOW I CAN HANDLE IT?

Well, yes, it is a skill; but the basic principles are easy enough to understand and follow. There are any number of excellent cookery books to help you acquire it: you'll find some suggestions below, and more in the Appendix.

What you need above all is a willingness to try, sharp knives, a

*see Appendix

good chopping board, and a loud timer to warn you when things are cooked.

Other essentials are good saucepans with lids, at least one really flat-bottomed heavyweight frying-pan, and two (or more) casseroles, also with lids.

The only other thing you must have is a respect for kitchen hygiene. Wash your hands before you start. Keep all surfaces clean. Never prepare salad vegetables or fruit with a knife or on a board that's been used for raw meat or fish, unless these have been well scrubbed first.

Cover all food when exposed. Put leftovers quickly into the fridge (but let them cool first).

This Isn't a Cookery Book – But It Does Contain Some Advice and Ideas to be Going on with

If you're an enthusiastic cook with a wide repertoire (particularly of vegetables), then you may want to skip this whole section.

But if, on the other hand, you have in the past relied heavily on packaged and processed foods (and three-quarters of the food bought in Britain today is in fact in processed form) then perhaps at this point you'll be reassured to find a little help and inspiration coming up.

COOKING FROM SCRATCH

VEGETABLES

This section starts by concentrating on vegetables, as you'll probably find that the important role they play in your Essential Diet is about to be the biggest change in the way you think about food. It certainly is for most people.

If you've done little vegetable cooking up to now, investing in a couple of good vegetarian recipe books makes good sense. Try *The*

Vegetable Epicure (Anna Thomas, Penguin, 1974); or any of Thorson's wide range of vegetarian cook books.

Meanwhile, here are a few basic suggestions.

The principle always with vegetables is to buy them as fresh as possible, cook them as briefly as possible, in as little water as possible, and to eat them as soon as possible.

They're ready when they still have a bite to them.

Most vegetables, of course, can also be eaten raw.

PREPARING VEGETABLES

Most young *root vegetables* only need scrubbing. Unless you know your carrots have been organically grown, you should peel these instead. Always eat potatoes in their skins, unless they're badly marked and damaged.

Older vegetables need peeling. They may then either be left whole, or cut into slices or chunks, or diced. Make sure to end up with pieces of roughly the same size, so that all the bits are cooked and ready at the same time. (It's easier to prepare large swedes by slicing them across, then peeling the slices, and afterwards cutting them as you want.)

Most root vegetables (but not potatoes), can be eaten raw: cut into sticks, shredded or grated.

GREEN VEGETABLES – AND SIMILAR

Green cabbage. Cut off the outer leaves (keep them and slice them for soup). Cut it in quarters. Slice off the core at an angle. Slice the cabbage (as coarse or fine as you wish) across the point of each quarter.

Treat *white or red cabbage* in the same way, but discard limp outer leaves.

Spring greens. Cut or tear out the centre stem. Roll up each leaf lengthways, and slice diagonally across.

Sprout tops. Hold at the stem end. Slice across and across until you reach the coarse base. Remove any baby sprouts and add to the tops.

Sprouts. Remove outer leaves if limp. Cut a cross on the base.

Spinach. If large, tear out centre stalks. (Hold both sides of the leaf firmly in one hand, and pull the stem sharply with the other.) Dump the leaves in a sinkful of water and woosh them gently around. Lift out in both hands and place in a large bowl (or double sink) while you run out the water and grit. Repeat until the spinach is grit-free.

Broccoli. Cut off and discard any woody base. Cut the stalk(s) off beneath the flowering head. Slice each stem lengthways into two or four, depending on its thickness.

Cauliflower. Either cut into four and slice out the core; or separate into florets.

Leeks. Cut off the root. Slice upwards through the centre, plunge into a deep jug of water and leave to rinse clean. Then slice into pieces. (Use the tender green as well as the white.)

Celery. Remove the strings from the coarse outside pieces. Scrub well if necessary.

All these vegetables can be added raw (shredded) to salads.

BEANS AND PEAS

Peas. Pod by pressing the end opposite the stalk, pulling the two halves apart, and running the thumb along the peas. New thin ones and old fat ones are both harder to shell.

Beans. Top and tail them (whether runner, French or bobby). If they need stringing along the sides, it may be enough to pull the string away with your knife as you top and tail. Otherwise, remove it with a potato peeler, or a special bean stringer. (More and more stringless beans are now appearing in the shops every year.)

Broad beans. If very young, cook whole. Otherwise, shell them.

SOME OTHER VEGETABLES

Marrow. Peel. Then either cut into rings and remove the centre seeds; or slice lengthways into two (and again scoop out the seeds); or cut into seed-free chunks.

Courgettes. Top and tail. Use whole, or slice.

Peppers. Cut out the stalk, and take out the inner membranes and seeds. Use whole, or slice.

Aubergines (eggplants). Top and tail and cut diagonally into slices.

Chinese leaves. Remove any limp outside leaves. Slice the amount you want diagonally across and leave briefly in water to refresh.

WHAT TO DO WITH YOUR VEGETABLES

Vegetables may be steamed, simmered, fried, casseroled, or eaten raw.

Steaming is an excellent way to retain taste and vitamins. Place the vegetables in a steamer in a pan over boiling water, and cover tightly with a lid. Make sure that the water just keeps on the boil.

It's difficult to give any timings as it depends on how finely the vegetables are cut and how young they are. Green vegetables can be done in minutes, while root vegetables can take half an hour or considerably longer.

Simmering is a quick, easy way of treating almost any vegetable.

Bring some water to the boil.

Put the vegetables in a saucepan. It's better to have a large-based pan which can accommodate all your vegetables in one layer, rather than a smaller deeper one. See that the vegetables nestle up as close to each other as possible, without any empty spaces around the edges.

Make sure the gas or electric ring is hot.

Then pour the boiling water onto the vegetables. If you're cooking root vegetables or green beans or peas, aim just to cover them. If cabbage or sprouts or similar green vegetables, pour only ½" (1 cm) or so into the pan. The water will go off the boil because the vegetables are cold. Wait for a moment until it comes to the boil again, then immediately turn the heat down. Add a pinch of salt and, if you wish, a small lump of butter or a teaspoon of olive oil.

If you're cooking root vegetables, you may now put on a lid to cover them and leave them to get on with it. (But keep an eye on them.)

If peas or beans, place a lid three-quarters on.

If cabbage etc, don't cover at all, but keep an even closer eye and stir once or twice to make sure it's not sticking.

With spinach, add only a tablespoon of water, or even none at all (there's usually enough water clinging to the leaves after washing), and keep turning the leaves gently in the pan.

With broccoli, cook the stems first in a little boiling water; then, when they're almost cooked, put the heads in the pan and pour on boiling water to just cover them; add a little salt; leave for a minute or two and drain immediately.

Be very careful not to overcook any vegetables. The time taken can vary from two – three minutes (cabbage) to as long as 45 minutes (swedes).

What you want to aim for ideally is for the cooking liquid to evaporate as the vegetables cook, so that all the goodness is retained with the vegetables, and not dissipated in the water. You can't always calculate this correctly; but, in any case, any liquid left can be added to soups.

NB A very watery vegetable like marrow is better not cooked in water at all, but steamed, fried or baked. If you're in a hurry, you can compromise by placing marrow rings or chunks in a pan covered with boiling water, seasoning and a good teaspoonful or more of oil and then cooking rather briskly, stirring occasionally, until all the vegetable is cooked and all the moisture has evaporated.

Frying You can fry many vegetables apart from the obvious ones like onions, tomatoes and mushrooms. *Stir-fried* vegetables are quick, easy, and nutritious. Use any vegetable or any combination.

Shred the vegetables fairly coarsely, or cut into matchstick-sized pieces. Heat a tablespoon or so of oil in either a wok or a deep frying-pan. When it's hot, but before it smokes, add the vegetables and stir round quickly as you keep the heat high enough to fry rather than simmer.

If you're cooking a mixture of vegetables, start with the ones that take longest, and add the others as you go along. Just before they're all cooked, add a good shake of soy sauce. (If you like to experiment with even stronger flavours, before you add the vegetables fry gently in the oil a little grated root ginger and crushed garlic.)

How to Sprout Beans etc

Sprouting beans, peas, grains etc. is child's play – and very economical. As if by magic, a couple of tablespoons of the basic ingredient grows within four or five days into a sizeable portion.

You can buy from health food shops a stack of plastic draining trays which makes it even easier, but all you really need is a large jar. Mung beans are perhaps the easiest of all to start with. You'll need 2–3 tbsp (depending on the size of the jar).

Soak them overnight. Rinse well, and place in your glass jar. Cover with either a piece of butter muslin, or of aluminium foil or plastic with holes poked in. Lay the jar on its side. There should be enough beans to spread in a thin layer along the side (now the base).

Place the jar somewhere dark and, if possible, warm.

In the evening, remove the top, pour on water, and drain off again. Replace the top and put the jar back. Repeat this morning and evening for 4–6 days. As the sprouts grow, each time you rinse them the shells will float free and rise to the surface. Remove them with a fork.

The sprouts will be ready when the roots are about 2″ (6 cms) long, and two pointed leaves are just beginning to appear.

If you don't want to eat them right away, rinse them well, and put in a covered jar in the fridge. They will keep for three or four days.

They're excellent as part of any salad; and they also make a valuable contribution to stir-fried vegetables (see below).

Many varieties of pulses and grains can be sprouted in this way; but always make sure that you use only those sold for human consumption, and not for planting; as these could have been chemically treated.

(See also *The Complete Sprouting Book*, by Per and Gita Sellman, Thorsons, 1984.)

The more vegetables you have, the longer they'll take, as you'll have to do them in batches. But each batch will take only 3–4 minutes.

Stir-fried vegetables like this make a meal on their own. (Or, if you wish, you can add e.g. sliced fish or kidney or liver or chicken.)

Casseroling Many vegetables can be cooked in a casserole. Obviously, it would be too expensive to put the oven on specially, but if you're planning to use it anyway it's simple to add vegetables to cook like this.

All you have to do is put a little butter or oil in the casserole; add the vegetables, seasoning, and perhaps a very little water; and put on a tight lid. They take two or three times as long to cook like this as simmering on the top, but they need little looking after. It's a good method for root vegetables, marrows, courgettes, peppers, aubergines etc, but don't use it for quick-cooking green vegetables.

DRIED BEANS AND SO ON

There are many different kinds of dried beans and pulses – haricot, butter, kidney, field, black-eyed, borlotti; brown and red lentils; green peas and chick peas; they're all easy to prepare, nutritious (they're rich in protein), and cheap. (You'll find them even cheaper if you get them unpackaged from shops which buy in bulk.)

They're basically all cooked and prepared in much the same way.

Pour the dried beans or whatever into a sieve, stir them around, and pick out any bits of grit you spot.

Cover them with boiling water and leave them to stand for an hour or so. Then rinse them, put them in a pan, add more boiling water to cover well, bring them properly to the boil, cover, and boil briskly for ten minutes. (This is particularly important for red kidney beans.)

Herbs and Spices

All herbs and spices add flavour and colour to any dish. They're particularly useful for ringing the changes with vegetables at boring times of the year.

Fresh herbs are best. Several of the most common are not hard to grow, even if you only have space for pots on your windowsill. At most times of the year you can at least buy parsley; and often continental parsley, coriander, and mint. Watercress can also be used in much the same way as a herb; as can mustard and cress.

To keep fresh bunches of herbs When buying them, make sure they're put in a bag with the stalks unbent. When you get them home, plunge them head down in a bowl of cold water and leave them for an hour or so. (This simultaneously revives them while washing off dirt and insects.)

Then stand them right side up in a jug of water, place an ordinary brown paper or plastic bag loosely over them so as to envelop both herbs and jug, and leave in the fridge or a cool larder. The herbs will keep fresh and green like this for a week or ten days.

To chop fresh herbs Strip off the leaves, or place the heads in a cup; then chop downwards with sharp scissors.

Dried herbs are a useful standby. Experiment. Try thyme with chicken, rosemary with lamb, oregano (the pizza herb) with cheese and tomato.

Spices are also better bought whole and freshly ground. If you buy them already ground – admittedly much easier – make sure it's from a shop which has a rapid turnover. (Old spices soon lose their savour.) Among the most useful are turmeric (not strong – adds a natural yellow colouring), paprika, ginger, coriander, cumin, nutmeg, cinammon.

Some seeds also combine happily with certain vegetables: try caraway with cabbage, or dill with turnip.

Add a bay leaf, a little garlic if you like, a good dash of oil, salt – about ½ – 1 level teaspoon per 8 oz (250 gms)* and pepper, some herbs or spices if you want, cover, and leave to simmer slowly. If you're worried about their digestibility, you can also add a dash of asafoetida or hing which you can find in Asian shops.

The time taken varies depending on the type of beans etc. and how long they've been stored. Red lentils are quickest – they can cook overall in 20–30 minutes; chick peas and some haricots are slowest, and take an hour and a half, or even two to three hours.

A pressure cooker is very helpful here. If you have one, check the instructions and times with your model.

Once cooked, all pulses can be used in various ways.

You can eat them:
    just as they are;
    or with any other permitted vegetables added (onions, mushrooms, tomatoes etc);
    or puréed and turned into soups;
    or strained, cooled, and shallow-fried;
    or crushed, spiced, and made into rissoles;
    or, when cold, served with a dressing, either on their own or plus other vegetables, as a salad;
    or squashed up, mixed with a little olive oil or tahini (a sesame seed paste), lemon, herbs or spices, and served as a dip or pâté.

*Adding salt while you cook beans is supposed to toughen them. I haven't found this to be so

MEAT

If you've been used to eating a lot of relatively 'convenience' meats – sausages, beefburgers, ham, luncheon meat – then to begin with you may find it takes a bit of thought and ingenuity to plan, shop for and cook just straightforward meat.

Prime quality cuts are expensive, and in general too dear for anything but special treats; but you can buy a small amount to use only as part of a much larger vegetable-based dish.

Pork or lamb chops or fillets, or any frying or grilling steak, need not simply be cooked in the piece. You can, for example, take the fillet, or the chop(s) minus the bones, and, with the fat trimmed, slice the meat thinly across the grain.

You can then either use the slices as they are, or cut them across and across again into matchsticks. Fry the slices quickly for 3–5 minutes (depending on the thickness of the slices), and then serve with vegetables and a sprinkle of lemon or chopped herbs or herb butter. Or fry the matchsticks as part of stir-fried mixed vegetables.

Cheaper cuts of meat, which need cooking for a much longer time, seem awkward to fit into a working day, but there ways are around this.

You can use a pressure cooker, and – depending on the meat – have a stew ready in 15–30 minutes. If you're an early riser, you can use a slow cooker and come back to a ready meal. Or you can cook a meal in the evening, cool it, put it in the fridge, and reheat it (thoroughly) the following day. This last is a good method to use with fatty cuts, such as stewing lamb. The fat will solidify on the top overnight in the fridge, and you can then lift it off.

Aim to have a hearty stew with plenty of vegetables, some cooked with the meat to add to the flavour.

Mince is so versatile that you probably already have several favourite ways of cooking it. Good lean mince will make your own beefburgers. Chopped fresh herbs are a tasty addition.

Fattier, lower grade mince needs longer cooking. Fry it gently first to release the fat, and then pour this away. Then add the stock (and vegetables or whatever), season it, bring it to the boil, and then simmer it gently (covered) for 1½ hours–2 hours.

Your butcher may be able to supply also minced lamb and minced pork. Some of the supermarkets also sell it, both fresh and frozen. This can help to give you the greater variety you're looking for. You can use either in much the same way as you can ordinary mince, though both texture and taste will be different.

Lamb's kidneys can be grilled whole. Both lamb's, pig's and ox kidneys can also be sliced (remove the core), and fried gently for a couple of minutes until they're cooked but still pinkish.

Ox liver should be casseroled. Pig's or lamb's liver can be fried. Again, the secret is to fry it gently and only for a short while, so that it's cooked but again pinkish (and not brown and hard) inside. One way to avoid over-cooking is to place the sliced liver in a small pan, pour boiling water over so as to just cover it, put on a lid, turn off the heat, and leave the pan for 5–10 minutes. Then take out the liver; shake off the water; and just heat it through gently in a little melted butter in a frying pan (turning once) for two or three minutes.

Frying Has Had a Bad Press

It's not so much frying in itself which is a bad idea, but frying things which soak up lots of fat or oil – and often doing this every day or even more than once a day.

Be as varied with your methods of cooking as you are with foods. Feel free to fry occasionally – but make sure it stops at that.

Always use the minimum of oil. You normally need only enough to prevent what you're cooking from sticking to the pan.

FISH

Fish is easy to prepare, quick to cook, and there's little waste.

It's surprising, then, that a lot of people are wary of buying it. If that's been true of you – be adventurous. You won't regret it. If you're fortunate enough to have a good local fishmonger, he'll both advise you and help with preparing and filleting fish.

There are basically three sorts of fish: *white fish, oily fish, and shellfish.*

Leaving shellfish for the moment, you can either buy fish whole (only practicable with smaller fish); in fillets (boneless); or cut into cutlets or steaks (with a bone).

All fish can be steamed (see vegetables), simmered (poached) – not generally a good idea, as most fish are so moist already – fried, grilled, or casseroled. Because all fish cooks so quickly, unless you're preparing an unusually large fish kept whole to feed a group of people, grillling or frying often makes most sense.

Pat the fish dry. If you're using frozen fish, it's best to defrost it thoroughly, drain off the moisture, and dry really well on a kitchen towel. You can dust it with seasoned flour (corresponding to your grain of the day); but – provided you have a good pan – you can also fry it without. Or grill it (brush the rack with oil first). Oily fish is good rolled in oatmeal.

You can serve your fish with lemon, or herb butter, or a puréed vegetable sauce.

Or you can marinate it before cooking (try leaving it beforehand for half an hour or so in a vinaigrette – see below), or cook it with spices.

Fish is very tolerant and very flexible.

Cold cooked fish is good in salad. So is tinned fish (read the labels). You can also use tinned fish as part of a hot fish-and-vegetable dish. Tinned tuna is particularly good for this, as it's a really solid fish.

SHELLFISH

Most shellfish is too expensive to be used except rarely, but even small amounts can be useful to add variety. Humble cockles, winkles and whelks are good with salad. Mussels, when in season, are still comparatively cheap. They're easy to do once you know how to clean them (scrub them well, and pick out the dead ones: they float). Consult a cookery book for full details.

How to Eat Fish

Some steer clear of fish because they dread getting entangled with all those bones. If this is really going to be a hang-up, stick with fillets or steaks until you get more confidence.

But a whole fish is no problem as long as you eat slowly and watch what you're doing. You can't just hack at it at random.

91

When you look at a whole round fish on your plate you'll notice that it has a stripe running right along the body. Cut gently right along this line until you touch the backbone which runs directly underneath. (A flat fish may not have so clear a mark, but otherwise it's basically the same. Follow the same procedure.) Then, with a fork, pull the flesh away in the direction of the diagonal bones. Ignore the fringey bits around the edges – they're full of tiny bones. Go carefully near the head, as there may be extra bones here too.

When you've eaten all the flesh on one side, pull the backbone upwards carefully away, and discard it. You can then comfortably eat the rest of the fish below.

POULTRY AND GAME

Chicken doesn't have to be fried or roast. It can also be casseroled, or cooked slowly on top of the cooker, with many different vegetables, herbs and spices to produce many different meals. The same is true of turkey – and duck; though most of us would probably prefer to cook this rare treat simply.

Venison can be treated in much the same way as similar cuts of beef. Stewing venison needs particularly long, slow cooking.

Rabbit can be fried, roast, casseroled, or cooked slowly on top of the cooker. Farmed rabbit is pale and rather bland; wild rabbit is darker and has a stronger, gamey flavour.

Game birds (pheasant, partridge etc) sold in supermarkets usually come packaged with their own instructions. If you buy from a butcher and are uncertain, ask for advice. Pigeon should be cooked slowly in a casserole: you need one bird per person.

GRAINS

Wholemeal bread
If you're *not* allergic to wheat, then wholemeal bread is an important staple. There are still parts of the country – especially in rural areas – where it's hard to come by. So here's a recipe. There's nothing tricky about it.

The quantities here are for one larger-than-1 lb loaf. It's simpler and more economical (as far as fuel consumption is concerned) to prepare and bake in two or three times this quantity. However, if you think you might be tempted to eat when you shouldn't (check again with p. x. above) then don't make more than you need.

1 lb (500 gms) plain wholemeal flour
1 tsp (5 ml) sugar
2 tsp (10 mls) dried yeast
2 tsp (10 mls) salt
about ⅓ pint (300 mls) lukewarm water
2 tsp (10 mls) oil

Dissolve the sugar in 3 or 4 tbsp of the warm (it should feel just warm but not at all hot when you put your finger in) water, and then sprinkle the yeast over the top. Leave the yeast, sugar and water in a warm place for 15 minutes. (The yeast uses the sugar to start fermenting.)

Then put the flour and salt in a large bowl. Make a well in the middle. Pour in the warm water, plus the yeast mixture (which should by now be frothing) and add the oil to the well. Now mix the liquid into the flour, first with a wooden spoon and then with one hand (first rub your hands lightly with oil). You need enough moisture for the resultant dough to leave the bowl clean, but still to be on the dry side rather than sticky.

Then take the ball of dough out of the bowl, and knead it on a floured board. Keep kneading for 5 or 10 minutes, until you can feel that it's elastic and all of the same texture throughout.

Put it into an oiled basin and cover losely with a piece of polythene or a damp tea towel. Leave it to rise. When it's risen to double its size, remove it from the basin, and knead it again briefly. Then leave it in a greased loaf tin (or make a ball and put it on a greased oven tray), and leave it to rise once more (with oiled polythene on top) until double its size.

Preheat your oven to 8 gas, 450°F, 230°C. Brush the top of the bread with milk, and bake in the centre of the oven for about 30 minutes. Test by removing the tin from the oven, turning out the loaf, and tapping the base. The bread is ready when the tapping sounds hollow.

Put the loaf on a wire tray to cool.

You can use the same recipe to make rolls.

Instead of bread, you can easily make *chapattis*. These use no yeast, and therefore need no time to allow for rising. Also, since they're 'baked' on top of the stove, they save on fuel costs.

8 oz (250 gms) wholemeal flour
1 tsp (5 ml) salt
about ⅓ pint (250 mls) water.

Sift the flour and salt into a large bowl. Make a well in the middle and pour in the water. Stir round first with a wooden spoon, and then with one oiled hand (as above) to make a dough. Put the dough on a floured board, and knead it briefly until it's elastic and an even texture. Then divide it into eight or ten pieces. Take each piece, and flatten it between your palms into a round; then use a rolling pin to roll each round out on a floured board into a thin circle.

When you're ready to eat them, 'bake' them one at a time on a lightly oiled frying pan (a griddle is ideal), for about 2–3 minutes each side. (After turning, press the sides down with a clean tea towel to encourage them to rise in the centre.) They should be cooked and faintly golden, but not dark brown.

BROWN RICE

Brown rice takes longer to cook than polished or par-boiled rice. It has a more positive, almost nutty flavour.

Measure one cupful. Shake this in a sieve and check to make sure there are no bits of grit. Then rinse well under running water.

Pour two cupfuls of boiling water into a wide-bottomed pan, and add 1 tsp (5 ml) sea salt and 1 tsp (5 ml) oil. Add the washed rice, and stir as it comes back to the boil again. Then immediately reduce the heat as low as possible, put on a tight lid, and leave it for about 30–40 minutes.

The rice is cooked when the water is absorbed, and a grain – when squeezed between finger and thumb – has no hard inner core, but is not squashy. Remove from the heat and leave to stand for at least another 5 minutes.

SALADS

Salads can be made with many different combinations of raw and cooked vegetables and fruit, plus – if wished – any of a whole range of protein and carbohydrate foods. Experiment with different combinations. Slice vegetables thinly, shred coarsely, or grate finely, to give a variety of textures.

Add a home-made salad dressing. A plain French vinaigrette is easy: 1 part wine vinegar to 3 of oil, plus a large pinch of salt, some pepper, and a little garlic and/or French mustard if you like. You can substitute lemon for the vinegar, and/or add freshly chopped herbs.

Not only can a well-planned salad be a main meal on its own; smaller salads are very handy for serving with or after (or indeed before) a larger course, to add nutrition, variety, and texture – and to fill in any odd gaps.

A short but very handy salad book, particularly useful with its ideas for winter, is *Salads For All Seasons*, by Josceline Dimbleby (A Sainsbury Cookbook, 1981).

EATING OUT

Sticking to your Essential Diet while eating out can present problems – especially if it involves eating somewhere with little choice, or in the company of others who may not understand why there are things you can and can't eat: particularly if those things keep changing from day to day!

The most likely places to be able to find and select what you want are wholefood or vegetarian restaurants, some ethnic restaurants, or the sort of pubs which cook fresh food and/or have a salad bar.

If there's nowhere like this handy or affordable, you may find you have no option, especially during the early days of your diet, but to prepare and take your own food to work – even if it means you have to be unsociable for a while.

Salt and Pepper

You'll find seasoning more interesting if you use sea salt and black pepper. You can buy special mills for grinding the salt and pepper. Or you can use Maldon sea salt flakes (rub them in your fingers) and buy ground black pepper (though it really does taste better if it's freshly ground).

Use salt sparingly. Research has shown that high salt levels (especially common in those who eat a lot of processed foods) have an adverse effect on health in general.

There's also the common observation that people who enjoy salted snacks (peanuts, crisps etc) tend to want to go on eating them. This can not only on its own contribute to a weight gain, but the salt makes eaters thirsty and turns them into drinkers – and what they drink (beer, cider, cola) also adds to their weight problem.

So use salt with circumspection. Never add it automatically at the table. Taste your food first. Unless something's gone wrong at the cook's end, you shouldn't need extra. As with sugar, all those shakes soon add up.

FORWARD PLANNING

As you see, there's nothing impossibly abstemious about your Essential Diet. And nothing (be honest, now) that you really can't tackle.

But what dieters often find it does require – as opposed to popping into a shop at the last moment – is a certain amount of organisation and forethought. Sitting down with a paper and pencil and working out menus beforehand can save a lot of wasted time and running around later.

But even if, overall, you do find that planning, shopping, and preparing meals (and possibly even eating them too) now take a larger chunk out of your time, remind yourself what your priorities are.

To lose (or gain) weight permanently – and hopefully to be healthier and happier than you were before. If extra time is the price you have to pay, then pay it as cheerfully as you can! Look round for other activities that you can cut down on to compensate. Cleaning windows. Reading the paper. Washing the car. Doing the crossword. Watching TV. . . .

CHAPTER 10

YOUR ESSENTIAL LIVING PLAN

At first sight, this chapter looks like a strange blend of opposites. The first half advises you to stir yourself up, while the second part suggests you calm yourself down.

But in fact, these prescriptions are complementary.

Too little physical activity, and too much stress – in its broadest meaning – both prevent the body from functioning as it's designed to. Each can affect the other. And both, in their different ways, can contribute to your weight problem.

HOW EXERCISE CAN HELP

Many people fall into a pattern of eating from habit, rather than from hunger. Very often it's a pattern that was established in childhood or in their teens, when indeed they probably *were* leading an active life and expending a lot of physical energy.

But as they grow into adults, and as their tastes change and they face more pressure both at work and home, there's often far less scope or time for really active pursuits. Their day-to-day and week-to-week life may demand almost no physical effort at all.

At the same time, they go on eating much the same food in much the same quantities – plus often the same kind of elevenses or teatime snacks. As a result, they begin to gain weight, and will go on gaining weight.

If in addition the food they're eating contains one or more allergens – which can be the case – then even in their late teens and twenties they may find themselves already headed for a life of recurrent or permanent weight problems.

The longer this pattern continues, the more persistent its effect, and the harder it is to alter it.

If this applies to you – and your Exercise column on p. 34 is sadly blank – then this is your opportunity to change.

As you follow your Essential Diet, you begin to break the habit form (and habit-forming) kind of eating; and at the same time you can alter your metabolism – the way and the rate at which your body utilises food – by increasing your level of physical activity.

How you choose to do it depends on your sort of life and your individual temperament.

Don't aim at some impossible target. Start with what you can readily fit in and cope with. Later, if you wish, you can progress gradually to something more demanding. Far better this way than work out a taxing schedule, fail to meet it, and then give up guiltily and in self-disgust.

If you think it would help to have the stimulus of a group activity, see what's available locally. In some parts of the country evening classes still offer facilities which compare very favourably with similar ones available privately. Be open-minded. It may be that something you've never considered before could in practice prove surprisingly attractive – tap-dancing or weight-lifting or t'ai chi.

Unless you're very fortunately placed, you're bound to have to take the money side into consideration. Swimming costs nothing but your entrance, costume, and drying your towel. Squash involves a (usually much higher) fee, plus racquet, the maintenance of good shoes, and washing and drying clothes. Start on something which will continue to be not only physically but financially within your possibilities.

SOLO SESSIONS

But of course it's perfectly possible – and considerably cheaper – to exercise on your own.

You don't have to have any elaborate equipment. All you need is bare feet or plimsolls, loose clothes, a very modest amount of space, a short period of time to yourself, and – the essential ingredient – the decision to do it rather than thinking about it.

Remember that any form of exercise should start with a warming-up period and finish with a cooling-down one. *Do not* – especially if you have taken no exercise for months or even years – suddenly jump up from your desk or cooker and set off on a two-mile jog. No matter how perfectly fit, no dancer would dream of leaping onto the stage stone-cold.

There are both books and tapes available to instruct and encourage. Don't buy the first one you see. Look at them, and decide which best covers the essential warm-up cool-down periods and offers a programme that you can actually keep to. Two recent books published by Thorsons, *Fully Fit In 60 Minutes A Week* (by Susanne O'Sullivan and Todd Easterbrook: one version for women, one for men), realistically plan for you to exercise three times a week.

This doesn't mean that you totally flop and do *nothing* on the other days. On the contrary. You should make a deliberate effort to introduce physical activity into your life whenever you can. Don't take the lift; if it's a manageable distance, use the stairs instead. Don't take a bus for three stops unless you're carrying a heavy load or pushed for time. Never take the car down the road to post a letter or pick up a magazine: walk instead.

Which brings us directly to *the* easiest form of exercise to incorporate into absolutely anybody's life. It's true it won't exercise every one of your muscles, and it's not glamorous. But it's totally do-able, you can start small and build up, it's not boring, and far from costing you it can actually save you money.

IT is a daily walk

If you set foot outside your door, walk briskly for ten minutes, turn round and walk briskly back again, you'll have walked a mile. Almost everyone, no matter how busy, can at some point in the day look at their watch or clock and say to themselves: 'Twenty minutes? I can spare twenty minutes.'

You don't have to go anywhere to do it, or even change your clothes (though it does make more sense to wear flat shoes than not). It sounds so little, and demands so little, that it hardly seems worth doing. But just as one hundred times nothing is nothing, but a hundred times £1 is £100, your daily short walks add up.

If after a while you step up your ten minutes to 15 (hardly any more), by the end of a week you'll have walked 10½ miles. If you previously never walked anywhere, that's just short of 550 extra miles a year!

Though you can walk any time, it's best to choose full daylight if you can. Natural light in itself is good for health. Not only does it supply vitamin D through the skin, recent research shows that it has a very positive effect both on the body's functioning and on mental attitudes.

Vary your walks as much as possible. If you're near public transport and can afford it, get a bus somewhere and walk back. Try setting yourself a daily different thing-to-look-at: chimneys or feet or trees or whatever. Chances are you'll very soon stop regarding it as a chore, and come to positively enjoy it. What's more, you'll soon realise how easily and quickly you can cover distances on foot you'd once have thought beyond you.

Cycling is another form of exercise which easily fits into many people's lives – and can again save money spent on transport. If you haven't cycled for years, the prospect can be daunting. Equip yourself with a bike in good order (it needn't be new: second-hand ones often turn up in local papers or on newsagents' cards, but any such purchases need to be well-checked), reflective band, good lights, and a strong chain and padlock. Make sure your brakes are always in good working order; then, at least to start with, keep to the back roads. Main roads are full of fumes anyway, and should always be avoided wherever possible.

The Less You Eat, the Better the Food Should Be

Those who are forced to lead a totally inactive life, through illness or injury, or in times of great stress or bereavement, need (and will in all probability want) comparatively little food. But that food should be of the highest quality: reduced to absolutely the essentials of the Essential Diet.

Tiny portions: but tiny portions of fresh fruit and vegetables, fresh meat and fish, wholemeal bread and brown rice (if tolerated). Definitely *not* sweetened foods, confectionery, and other non-food 'foods' which destroy the appetite, mean that real food is not taken, and deprive the body of essential nutrients. Many people can trace the start of their weight problems to just such episodes in their lives.

After a wary start, in all probability you'll find yourself actually relishing the experience – and pleased to realise how much money you can save.

Even a gentle exercise programme which includes either walking or cycling (or both) often has a beneficial effect not only on metabolism but also on mood. It's harder to be consistently depressed while your body is moving into a higher gear, and your activities are taking you out and about.

This is a modest example of the close relationship between physical activity and certain aspects of stress.

MIND AND BODY

People aren't divided into neat little packages of mind and body – each totally separate. What goes on in their bodies affects how people feel and think. And how people feel and think can affect how they function physically.

If you answered *yes* to question 19, then this could have a significant connection with the possible development of food allergies.

It's often been observed that some people under stress eat 'for comfort', while others completely lose their appetite. Apart from this apparently direct relationship, there is another. Specialist doctors have noted that certain individuals under stress become allergic either to the foods they enjoy and eat regularly, or to those they begin to refuse to eat.

It's not the stress itself that directly causes their food-related and weight-related problems (though it may look like it); but the fact that the stress acts as a trigger for the whole mechanism.

Under stress, the body can no longer cope with foods that are harmful to it. The consequent weight gain (or weight loss) may therefore not be due simply to someone eating too much (or not enough), but may arise from a much more complex chain of affairs.

'Stress', in this context, means any situation which puts unusual – and often prolonged – strain, mental or physical, on any individual. It can include bereavement, pregnancy, infectious illness (particularly glandular fever, or something which looks like glandular fever but isn't), problems over work or money, redundancy, and any kind of difficulties in family or personal relationships.

If you noticed that your weight problems (and perhaps other symptoms too) began during or shortly after a period of stress, then, again, this is a convincing indication that food allergies could be at least part of your difficulties.

So, in addition to sorting out your diet stage by stage, it makes sense to start from the other end as well: to try to remove or reduce the cause of stress if at all possible, and – when it isn't – to adopt positive and non-destructive methods of dealing with it.

Don't be too proud to seek help.

Feel free to talk to friends or relatives. Speak out about your worries, thoughts, fears. It can be a help even to write them down, get them out of your head, put them down where you can see them and start to work on them. Don't feel you always have to conceal problems or pretend. If you're troubled or worried, explain. Give others a chance to support you.

If you have a religious faith, talk your situation over with your priest or other members of your congregation.

Your GP may be able to advise you. In some areas, he/she can put you in touch with counsellors.

The Marriage Guidance Council too has trained counsellors to listen (though there are waiting lists in many areas); you'll find your local number in the phone book.

Or ring the Samaritans: they're not there just for the totally desperate, but also to provide an ear for those trying to cope with heavy burdens.

If your wider problem (or your family's problem) is also connected with any particular illness, you may well find there's a nationwide association that can help. Ask your GP; or your local library; or write to the advice page of a women's magazine.

Classes in yoga or meditation can also help. Enquire at your local evening institute.

There are also many supportive books available. Among others, Thorsons and Sheldon Press have particularly comprehensive lists. Send a sae for their catalogues.

None of this means that your A-Diet won't work unless you get your whole life sorted out first. It's simply acknowledging the truth that you are a whole person, and that it's by recognising this wholeness that you'll be best able tackle your diet – and to solve your weight and other health problems.

There is of course more to life than diet, exercise and coping with stress – a whole vital area which is outside the scope of this book.

So it's worth mentioning here that many dieters who successfully sort out their allergic problems are delighted (and astonished) to discover that they also release in themselves a positive and creative approach that's quite new to them.

More than one has explained: 'It's as though before I was always living in a mist;' or – like Jill Cooper – said: 'My whole personality has changed – for the better.'

Children and teenagers in particular often find marked benefits both at school and in their social life. Doctors have observed that 'learning difficulties in an otherwise bright child' may be connected with allergy, and clear up once the individual allergens are sorted out. The increased confidence resulting from the development of hitherto underused abilities spills over into their relationships with others.

The change in successfully diagnosed allergics is permanent. As one recently divorced single parent put it: 'I've been able to tackle a whole range of things I'd never have dreamed of doing before. What I've achieved so far mightn't be world-shaking, but it's important to me. And I could no more have done that before than I could fly.'

So, with the message of this chapter to encourage you, full speed ahead with your Essential Diet – and your Essential Living Plan!

CHAPTER 11

YOUR ESSENTIAL DIET DIARY

The first stage of your Essential Diet runs for eight days. If you would feel happier doing it for longer before drawing any conclusions, then be sure to continue keeping accurate notes of what you observe. Either use a notebook set aside for this purpose, or attach any separate sheets of paper firmly to this book: you may need this record later.

The meals this time are not broken down into their separate elements – though of course you'll continue to bear these in mind.

Weigh yourself as before, morning and evening.

Note down any *symptoms*. Don't forget to add when they stop as well as when they start.

You may well find your moods more changeable than ever before. Be sure to chart these carefully under *How you feel*.

Your *Exercise* column will probably have a lot more in it than during your AYAN period – and your *Exposure to chemicals* considerably less.

If earlier you began to associate symptoms or weight changes to specific *Happenings*, see if you can repeat these during the next eight days. Clearly, this doesn't mean starting a quarrel purely for research purposes! But you could, for example, aim to re-visit a restaurant or call again on the same group of relatives.

Above all, during this period, aim to enjoy your diet. Be positive. Like what you are eating – don't lament what you aren't.

If you find yourself eyeing the fridge wistfully, remove yourself from its presence. Walk, ride, phone, bath, paint, sweep, saw, chop. . . . anything but sit around fretting and drooling!

Remind yourself that any pangs will fade as days go by. And that patience and perseverance *will* win the prize.

DAY ONE

BREAKFAST

MIDDAY

EVENING

ANY EXTRAS

WEIGHT AM PM

EXERCISE

ANY SYMPTOMS

HOW YOU FEEL

EXPOSURE TO CHEMICALS

HAPPENINGS

DAY TWO

BREAKFAST

MIDDAY

EVENING

ANY EXTRAS

WEIGHT AM PM

EXERCISE

ANY SYMPTOMS

HOW YOU FEEL

EXPOSURE TO CHEMICALS

HAPPENINGS

DAY THREE

BREAKFAST

MIDDAY

EVENING

ANY EXTRAS

WEIGHT AM PM

EXERCISE

ANY SYMPTOMS

HOW YOU FEEL

EXPOSURE TO CHEMICALS

HAPPENINGS

DAY FOUR

BREAKFAST

MIDDAY

EVENING

ANY EXTRAS

WEIGHT AM PM

EXERCISE

ANY SYMPTOMS

HOW YOU FEEL

EXPOSURE TO CHEMICALS

HAPPENINGS

DAY FIVE

BREAKFAST

MIDDAY

EVENING

ANY EXTRAS

WEIGHT AM PM

EXERCISE

ANY SYMPTOMS

HOW YOU FEEL

EXPOSURE TO CHEMICALS

HAPPENINGS

DAY SIX

BREAKFAST

MIDDAY

EVENING

ANY EXTRAS

WEIGHT AM PM

EXERCISE

ANY SYMPTOMS

HOW YOU FEEL

EXPOSURE TO CHEMICALS

HAPPENINGS

DAY SEVEN

BREAKFAST

MIDDAY

EVENING

ANY EXTRAS

WEIGHT AM PM

EXERCISE

ANY SYMPTOMS

HOW YOU FEEL

EXPOSURE TO CHEMICALS

HAPPENINGS

112

DAY EIGHT

BREAKFAST

MIDDAY

EVENING

ANY EXTRAS

WEIGHT AM PM

EXERCISE

ANY SYMPTOMS

HOW YOU FEEL

EXPOSURE TO CHEMICALS

HAPPENINGS

113

CHAPTER 12

TAKING STOCK

Most Essential Dieters will, after the first eight days, find themselves in one of the following categories.

If you seem to fall evenly between two, continue for at least another eight days; or until you feel more confident about the conclusions you can draw. Otherwise, pick the one which you feel on balance is more likely to apply to you, and carry on from there.

1. You end up this period with a marked weight loss (or gain – whichever you were aiming for).

You've been symptom-free, and indeed feel unusually well.

You've been agreeably stable and even-tempered.

Then the Essential Diet, just as it stands, is right for you.

You may simply be benefiting from the removal of sugar and refined flour from your diet. And/or your body may have previously been reacting to chemicals and additives, and, free of this overload, can now cope. And/or, thanks to your increased activity, your metabolism has been altered for the better.

But it remains possible that your weight change is at least partly due to the removal (or reduction) of items to which you are – if only mildly – allergic.

So now that you've found a diet that suits you, be prepared to carry on with it indefinitely. As long as you continue to gain (lose) weight and to be well, it's wise not to tamper with it at all. Keep up the variety. Don't be tempted to start eating restricted items more often.

After at least three months (six is better), you can, if you wish, cautiously try – for example – eating bread (still wholemeal) rather more often. (After all, if you *can* eat it, it's an excellent food.) Or you may want to be able to use more eggs, or reintroduce orange or apple juice. (See p. 185 before you start.)

But be alive to any subsequent changes, and be ready to cut down again. Be sure to go on avoiding eating monotonously.

You won't go on and on gaining (losing) weight, by the way. Your appetite and your consumption will balance each other. You'll arrive at a weight which is right for you, and you'll then stop.

2. Over this period you've lost (or gained) weight, but without noticing any abrupt day-to-day rises or falls. It doesn't matter whether the overall gain (or loss) was as little as 1 or 2 lbs. What is significant is that it's happened.

You've been relatively, but not completely, symptom-free. You've also been reasonably equable and well-balanced – no uncalled-for temper tantrums or fits of depression. (*Justified* mood changes don't count.)

Then keep on this diet indefinitely. It obviously suits you and – provided you're careful to follow the guide-lines, it's likely to go on suiting you.

Don't take liberties with it though. It remains possible that you're allergic to something you're continuing to eat (or drink). But as long as you're varying your diet and not eating repetitively, than you'll go on being able to tolerate any such problem items.

Don't try to increase the frequency of any restricted foods for six months; possibly earlier, if you completely cease to have any symptoms at all.

3. Your weight stayed the same throughout. You noticed no marked ups and downs, and you neither lost nor gained.

Your symptoms either cleared completely, or noticeably decreased. Your temperament either remained unchanged, or became calmer.

The decrease of symptoms is an indication that you're likely to be on the right track. Sometimes a resultant weight change is slow to follow.

Keep going on this diet for another eight, 16 or 24 days.

After this interval, you may find you have moved into category 1 or 2. If so, follow the appropriate directions.

But if, on the other hand, you've noticed no further change, then it's time to turn to Chapters 13 and 14 and plan your next move.

4. Your weight, though ending up much the same as when you started, showed marked rises and falls in between.

You had as many symptoms as before, though of much the same kind, and no more severe.

You experienced mood changes, without any real cause.

Then you're being affected by certain currently permitted elements in your Essential Diet. Perhaps by now you already have a strong suspicion about what's causing your trouble. If so, carry on with the diet as before, for another eight or 16 days.

Does the pattern then repeat itself? Do you notice mood changes which correspond with physical symptoms? And also with weight changes?

As with your AYAN Diary, check back, first through 24 hours, and then 48 hours. Can you relate any symptom or weight change, on more than one occasion, to the same specific foods?

If you finally feel you may have tracked down your suspects, then move on to Chapters 13 and 14, continuing to bear this in mind.

CHAPTER 13

ALLERGY – SOME CAUSES AND EFFECTS

So your answers to the quiz showed that you might indeed be food-allergic.

Your days on your Essential Diet have helped to confirm this.

And yet – in your heart of hearts – you still don't genuinely believe it's possible?

Well – you'll be interested to know most of those who go on to confirm that they *are* allergic start by feeling just as you do now. Just as reluctant to accept that they may have to make pretty basic changes in the way they eat – and live. Just as unwilling to face giving up precisely those foods (and drinks) they most enjoy.

And of course, what makes the whole idea even harder to accept is that it's often the foods (and drinks) that everyone thinks of as particularly healthy which cause most problems.

Why?

Why should some individuals be unable to tolerate bread, milk, oranges, potatoes, cheese, tomatoes – or even apples, cabbage or carrots?

At present the unsatisfactory answer is that there *is* no answer – or at least no one answer. Here are some thoughts which may have a bearing on the question.

1. Some individuals are born with a fixed allergy (as defined by orthodox immunologists – see p. 19) to one or more specific foods: something as ordinary as cow's milk, or as exotic as green peppers. They will never be able to tolerate whatever-it-is; it will always affect them right through their lives.

2. Some – a much larger number – develop allergies – perhaps as a result of eating (drinking) whatever-it-is in unusually large quantities. But, at present, it's impossible to sort out effect from cause. Do they become allergic because they eat (drink) excessive amounts? Or do they eat (drink) excessive amounts because they're allergic (addicted)?

3. Some doctors, such as Dr Richard Mackarness (author of *Not All In The Mind*), consider that human beings are basically designed to eat a primitive 'Stone Age' diet: essentially meat, fish, vegetables, fruit, nuts. They are only partially (and in individual cases, not at all) adapted to eating later 'farmed' foods, such as grains and dairy products.

4. Others would add that different peoples have traditionally eaten different diets. Now, with the import of many 'exotic' foods, individuals are regularly eating foods that their ancestors would only rarely have encountered. Again, these doctors believe that some cannot cope with such a diet on an everyday basis.

5. Many doctors believe that food allergies are primarily due to damage to the immune system, caused above all by harmful chemicals: present in the air, in the soil, in the water, and in medically prescribed drugs. These, absorbed into the individual's system, alter and distort the way it functions.

6. This pollution also, they contend, creates a 'perversion of appetite'. This is what causes certain individuals to eat abnormally. There is no accurate awareness of hunger or of satisfaction of hunger.

7. Some allergies appear to be triggered off by viral infections; or by antibiotics.

8. Some allergies aren't 'allergies' at all – though they may produce very similar allergic-type reactions. They are in fact *direct* responses to chemicals sprayed on, grown with, or added to a whole range of foods.

Although there are certainly plenty of indications that more and more people are becoming food-allergic, yet there's also evidence that it's not only a twentieth century problem. Fabienne Smith, herself a 'universal reactor' (allergic to virtually everything), has documented the existence of allergy in a number of literary and historical figures.

So, if you too turn out to be allergic to foods and/or chemicals, you're in good company. It looks as though Charles Darwin and Lady Hamilton – among others – may have been among those similarly affected!

But today, unlike those others in the past, you can now actually discover the cause of your problems. Once you acknowledge to yourself that food allergy *may* be the answer, you're well on the way to identifying your own particular food enemies.

And when you do, you can eliminate them.

It's far too late for you to pick different parents and so be born less sensitive. You can't do anything to change what's happened to you up till now. But the message is that you *can* do something about your allergies from this time on. Indeed, having got so far, you're already well on the way.

One of the beauties of this approach is that it doesn't matter how long you have, unknowingly, been suffering from food allergies, or how old (or young) you are: once you identify and remove the things that are harming you, your recovery – your return to 'normality' – can be rapid.

As an extra bonus, you'll find that you sort out not only your weight problems, but other symptoms that – before you picked up this book – you doubtless never dreamed could be connected.

Because people who weigh too much (or too little) as a result of reactions to foods (or chemicals) almost always have other health problems as well.

As you've already gathered, when you track down your problem foods (and/or chemicals), you'll not only reach your proper weight. You'll find your symptoms vanishing at the same time.

WHAT SORT OF SYMPTOMS?

Almost any symptom you like to name *could* be caused by allergies.

Any single one of these could alternatively, of course, be caused by something else.

But there's a clear indication that allergies may be to blame *if*:
neither GP nor specialist can identify any other actual *cause*;
your symptoms don't respond to any treatment;
or they keep coming back as soon as a treatment course is over;
or they've persisted over a number of years (perhaps even most of your life).

So here's a list of the most common of such symptoms*

Aches (of All Kinds)

Acne

Aggression

Anxiety

Arthritis

Asthma

*For further information on the links between diet and allergically-caused illness, see *The Allergy Connection*, Barbara Paterson, Thorsons, 1985.

Bed-Wetting
Bilious Attacks
Bladder Problems
Blood Pressure (High or Low)
Bowel Problems (IBS: Irritable Bowel Syndrome)
Bronchitis
Catarrh
Colic
Colitis
Constipation
Crohn's Disease
Cystitis
Depression
Diarrhoea
Earache (and Other Ear Problems)
Eczema
Exhaustion
Eye Problems (Conjunctivitis, Dark Rings, Grittiness etc.)
Headaches
Hives (Urticaria)
Indigestion
Insomnia
Irritability
Migraines
Menstrual Problems
Mood Changes
Nausea
Nightmares
Runny Nose, or Blocked Nose
Panic Attacks
Period Problems
Personality Changes
Pre-Menstrual Tension
Rashes
Rheumatism
Skin Problems
Sleep Problems
Stomach Problems
Excessive Sweating
Sore Throats
Tonsillitis

Thrush
Ulcers
Vomiting

How the A-Diet Can Help Other Sufferers Too

Many people who suffer from the symptoms on the previous pages (and from others as well), but *without* the extra warning of weight problems, may in fact be reacting to undiagnosed food and chemical allergies.

The clues are the description of the *type* of symptoms just given on p. 121; and the likelihood of allergy, worked out from the answers to the quiz on p. 21.

The A-Diet which will cause you to lose both your weight problems *and* your symptoms may also help others who have the symptoms without the weight problems. Exactly the same procedure should be followed, starting with the AYAN Diary.

The only difference is that tea, coffee, alcohol and chemicals may play a larger role. Anyone without weight problems who suspects their symptoms could be due to food or chemical allergies should read in particular the piece on p. 201 and Chapter 18 on p .198.

And now gird yourself to discover, as so many already have, that with so much to gain, it's worth the sacrifice – even of your favourite cereal or cheese or chips.

CHAPTER 14

ELIMINATION DIETS AND HOW TO HANDLE THEM

By now, hopefully, you'll have a good idea which foods and drinks you most suspect. The next move is to cut them out of your diet; either one at time, or in groups, or altogether in one fell swoop.

You'll find further help with selecting the right elimination diet for you below in Part 3. But here, to start with, is some essential background information.

PART 1. GENERAL PRINCIPLES

Whichever elimination diet you go on to select, the basic method remains the same.

You continue on your Essential Diet, and follow your Essential Living Plan, but you restrict your foods/drinks still further – depending on which version it seems to make best sense to adopt.

You cut out *completely* from your diet the food(s) or drink(s) you suspect of causing your problems. *That means completely. You mustn't have so much as a sip or a mouthful of whatever-it-is.*

The normal recommended time for an elimination diet is five days. This is almost always long enough for children and teenagers. However, the older you are, and the longer you've been exposed to whatever-it-is, then the longer you may need to abstain.

For example, if you're in your forties, and you've been eating bread every day for most of your life, then you may need to cut out all wheat for seven or eight days – or even longer – before you notice any change.

Ten days is normally the longest period necessary. If by then you've noticed no differences at all, then it's highly improbable that whatever you've been leaving out has any effect on you.

125

Any elimination diet demands organisation beforehand.

If you think you might be tempted by the sight or smell of the food or drink you're testing, then take it out of your fridge or kitchen and give it away. If you're living with family or friends, explain what's happening and try to get their co-operation – it isn't easy to resist if you're dreaming of bread and a loaf appears in the bread-tin.

Make sure you have plenty of a variety of other foods available. Stock up particularly on suitable alternatives.

Don't plan to begin an elimination diet at a busy or difficult time. If it's at all possible to take a week off work, do so. Don't make any social commitments which put any extra strain on you.

Fill in your Elimination Diet Diary for at least five days. If by then the results are not conclusive; and/or you'd previously been eating/ drinking the suspect item(s) for many years, then continue for another 1 – 5 days. (Make sure you keep the information safely either in a separate notebook, or on sheets firmly attached to this book.)

WHAT DO THE RESULTS SHOW?

After the initial elimination period (whether five, or six – 10 days) look back at the overall picture your diary now shows.

YOU'LL FIND THAT YOUR EXPERIENCES FIT INTO ONE OF FOUR CATEGORIES

1. *No change* Apart from the inconvenience of changing your pattern of eating, you notice no difference at all. Your weight hasn't changed. Your symptoms – if any – haven't altered either for the better or the worse. You feel much the same as usual.

Then you can be reasonably sure that the particular food(s) or drink(s) you're testing are safe for you.

Withdrawal Symptoms

As mentioned earlier on p. 116, you may already have suffered from withdrawal symptoms during your Essential Diet.

On any of the more restricted elimination diets which follow, the chances of withdrawal symptoms increase. However, it's impossible to predict for any individual whether he or she will have any at all: or, if so, whether they'll be mild or severe. Many people can give up foods which are subsequently proved harmful without more than a mild regret or a few days of feeling a bit under the weather.

If you do get withdrawal symptoms, they will be at their worst during the first one to three days, fading or changing after that until they disappear altogether.

The Symptoms May Include:

headaches
pains in the back of the neck, thighs, lower back
extreme sleepiness, or insomnia
nausea, vomiting
palpitations
diarrhoea
sweating
depression, or mental changes
difficulty in focussing
'just feeling lousy'
exacerbation of your own normal symptoms

If you do have withdrawal symptoms, don't take any pain-killers, indigestion remedies etc. Remind yourself that these are a very good indication that the foods you're eliminating are harmful to you; and also that they will fade away.

However, if you're one of the small but important minority who find extreme difficulty in elimination diets, go back to replacing whatever you've been leaving out, and seek specialist advice (see p. 212).

2. *A withdrawal curve PLUS* You feel low the first few days, and may even suffer from marked withdrawal symptoms, headache, or deeply depressed. Then you begin to notice a gradual improvement, followed by a marked improvement. Some or even all your previous symptoms disappear.

Your weight drops (or rises) considerably.

Then you can be positive that you're allergic to one at least of the food(s) or drink(s) you're testing.

3. *Weight change alone* You don't feel a great deal of difference between the way you felt before and during the elimination diet; *but* by the end you notice a marked change in your weight.

Then you can be reasonably certain that you're allergic to one at least of the food(s) or drink(s) you're testing.

4. *Vanishing symptoms* You notice no weight change after the first week on the diet; *but* you feel ill during the first few days, and gradually improve thereafter. Previous symptoms you suffered from diminish or disappear.

Then, again, you can still be reasonably confident that you're allergic to one at least of the food(s) or drink(s) you've been testing. (A weight change may well follow later. It can take as long as two or more weeks to show itself.)

WHAT NEXT?

If you answered *yes* to question 1, then you can resume eating normally the food(s) or drink(s) you've just been testing. Proceed to the next most suspect item(s). Check again with the suggestions below.

If you answered *yes* to 2, 3 or 4, then you have two choices.

1. Are you satisfied now that whatever you've been cutting out was contributing to your weight problems (and possibly other symptoms)? And are you happy simply to continue leaving out those food(s)/drink(s)?

Then there's no need to test it/them any further.

Keep following the same diet, and don't stop monitoring your progress. (You may like to use some of the spare pages at the back for this purpose.)

Yes – it is a bit of a chore, but it's a sound idea to maintain such a record. Noting your steady improvement gives you a welcome boost

– and you'd be surprised how quickly you can forget the information you're jotting down. It may well be useful to you later.

If you still feel that there may be other foods involved, then of course you can go on to eliminate these too. You can either do this straight away, or you can wait until you've become more at home with your present revised diet.

After you've been on your new diet for at least six months, it may be possible to try reintroducing foods. This needs thinking about. Turn to the piece on p. 130.

2. You may want to *prove* whether or not you are indeed allergic to whatever you've been testing. You do this by carefully reintroducing your suspect items (details below).

If you've been testing *only one item,* and answered *yes* to 2 or 3, the only real justification for reintroducing your suspect food/drink is to convince yourself – or perhaps your family or friends – by your reactions that allergy really is involved.

As all the evidence of your diet already indicates that this is likely to be the case, any such reactions could be severe. So before doing this, weigh up carefully whether it's likely to be worth while.

If you've been testing only one item, answered *yes* to 4, and miss whatever-it-is considerably, then you might feel it worth while risking reactions to discover whether or not this does indeed affect you – or whether the reduction of symptoms you've noticed might perhaps be pure coincidence.

But the most common reason for reintroducing and testing foods is to discover if, out of a group eliminated at the same time, any are in fact harmless.

If you've been testing *several items together* (e.g. all dairy products, or all grains), then reintroducing individual items one by one is the only way of deciding whether all, or only some, are harmful to you.

If you don't mind continuing to leave the whole lot out (or at least leaving them out for at least 3 – 6 months), then again there's no point in experimenting with reintroducing them.

But if you want to find out if there are any you can safely eat/drink, then reintroducing them under controlled conditions is the only way to discover this for yourself.

REINTRODUCING FOODS/DRINKS

The procedure is the same every time.

You may reintroduce the suspect item as soon as your withdrawal symptoms (if any) have cleared, and you feel well. This can be as early as the sixth day after you started your elimination diet; or any day after that.

Don't try reintroduction if you *don't* feel well. If you've already got a headache or indigestion, it will be impossible to decide later whether or not your reintroduced food is adding to your problems.

Aim to test your food/drink at midday.

Children on Elimination Diets

It's advisable to use elimination diets on children only during holiday periods. That way, you can both keep an eye on results, and help your son/daughter through any bad withdrawal periods.

Shortly before your test, take your pulse (*not* immediately after you've been rushing around or doing anything strenuous: while you're in a sitting-down or resting state.)

How to Take Your Pulse

Place the first two fingers of one hand just below the base of the thumb of the other hand. Use a digital watch or clock or any watch with a second-hand. Count the number of beats in one minute.

Then eat or drink a reasonable amount of the suspect item: two slices of bread, or a glass of milk, or a whole orange. Don't eat or drink anything else at the same time, or you risk confusing the issue.

Take your pulse again 1) 20 minutes, 2) 40 minutes and 3) 60 minutes after eating or drinking your challenge portion.

Note down any symptoms, and the time at which you observed them.

Continue noting any symptoms for a further 48 hours.

If your reactions are severe, you may take one of the remedies on p. 71.

130

A change in your weight, and/or an increase in your symptoms, both indicate that you're allergic to what you're testing. A rise (or, occasionally, a fall) in your pulse rate of over 10 beats per minute helps to confirm this. (However, it's possible to have a weight change and/or an increase in symptoms without any accompanying pulse change. Any change in your weight or symptoms is more significant.)

If you're still uncertain, leave the food/drink out for a further week or two, and then re-test again.

If you've had no adverse reactions, and you feel perfectly well by midday the following day, then you may go on to reintroduce another food. Follow exactly the same procedure. (Some foods, grains in particular, demand longer intervals between testing. You'll find this noted under the specific elimination diets.)

Repeat with different items as often as necessary.

If you do find yourself in a muddle at any point, break off the reintroduction and testing altogether. Go back to the version of your Essential Diet which you believe is safe, or relatively safe, for you; and leave further testing for a while.

Reasons to Keep Going

As you probably know from experience, changing your way of eating (and living) is always a struggle. An elimination diet can be particularly stressful, as it often asks you to give up just the foods and drinks that you most enjoy.

So stop to remind yourself of what you've already achieved – and why it's worth while to keep going.

You want to be and look the sort of person you know you really are.

You want to feel fit and healthy – not always a bit off colour.

You want to feel positive and at peace with yourself – neither apologetic nor aggressive.

You're tired of diets which either don't work at all, or don't work permanently.

You wish you didn't have to feel guilty when you're *not* on a diet.

You never want to count calories again.

You're fed up with feeling a failure.

And you're prepared to give yourself a chance.

PART 2 WHERE TO FIND HELP

You may feel, like many others, that life would be easier if you had some support – someone to call on over the next few weeks: for advice, or practical help, or for psychological support if nothing else.

Your GP may be able to help, particularly if you've been consulting him or her in the past over your weight problems and/or your symptoms.

Today, several hundred GPs are now members of various organisations concerned with the effects of the diet on health, such as the British Society for Clinical Ecology, the British Society for Nutritional Medicine, the McCarrison Society, and the Society for Environmental Therapy etc.

Many others, while not formally belonging to any specific group, are becoming increasingly interested in this approach.

Because of the pressure on the average GP's time, and also because of the frequent hostility of patients to the idea that what they eat and how they live can affect their health, doctors frequently wait for their patients to approach them to broach this idea, rather than the other way round.

So do start with a visit to his/her surgery.

Doctors who are either knowledgeable already, or prepared to be open-minded, can help with constructive advice, support during withdrawal symptoms (if any), and even prescriptions for helpful vitamin and mineral supplements (though the NHS situation in this respect keeps changing).

Your GP may also be able to refer you to an *NHS specialist or clinic* This depends on the area in which you live. There are currently very few specialists available, and only a handful of allergy clinics which offer advice on food and elimination diets (see also p. 213); however, these numbers are growing all the time.

If you find your GP incredulous or even hostile to the whole idea of either food or chemical allergies, don't lose heart. Remember, as mentioned earlier* that during their training doctors are taught very little about either nutrition or allergy, and that although important papers have been published in the medical journals most GPs are too snowed under by work and words to have time to catch up.

There are still steps you can take.

There are also now a score or so of doctors, most of whom have

*p. 17.

worked in this field for several years, who run *private specialist clinics*. It's sometimes possible to claim for such treatment through private health insurance.

It is of course not easy to discover such doctors. Your GP – if sympathetic, though inexperienced – may be able to refer you. Otherwise, you can seek help from Action Against Allergy or the National Society for Research into Allergy; or, if it's for your child, from the Hyperactive Children's Support Group.* The problems of over/underweight and hyperactivity overlap, and therefore the same doctors can advise on both.

Doctors prefer a GP's referral, but most will not refuse to see you if your GP is adamantly against this, or you would prefer not to have to ask.

There are also *allergy clinics* run by lay advisers who may not be medically qualified, but have very considerable experience. They too may be able to offer valuable support and advice. It is, obviously, wise to make enquiries before contacting any of these. Again, your GP may be able to tell you more (even if unofficially); or if you have a reputable local health food shop, you could try asking there.

Alternative practitioners may also be another source of help. However, this depends on the individual's knowledge and experience. An acupuncturist or a homeopath may not *necessarily* be able to help; but – given the right background – often they can.

Private specialists, privately run clinics, alternative practitioners – all cost money. If, like most of us, you have little to spare, then what can you do?

Many on elimination diets find help from *support groups*, composed of individuals who are either allergic themselves or have allergic children. They meet regularly to exchange recipes and hints, and between meetings offer each other encouragement, support, and practical advice. Some buy organic foods, or food replacements, in bulk; or invite speakers; or even raise money for research.

If your doctor is sympathetic, he may know whether a group exists locally. Enquiries at your library or health food shop may produce results. Otherwise, contact AAA, the NSRA or HCSG.

*See p. 219 for addresses

TESTING AND DIAGNOSIS

Private clinics can also offer alternative methods of testing for diagnosis and treatment. See below, p. 212.

All this doesn't mean that it's impossible for you to tackle your A-Diet on your own. This certainly isn't so. It's just that – as with many diets – a little psychological hand-holding at the right moment can make a lot of difference. And fellow-company in hard times is always welcome!

Vegetarians and Elimination Diets

It's difficult for vegetarians to undertake elimination diets, since they may need to cut out either grains, dairy products, or both. Doctors suggest either a very careful and varied – though restricted – diet, or a fast on spring water, or a semi-fast on permitted fruit.

PART 3 WHICH ELIMINATION DIET FOR YOU?

1. Did your AYAN Diary show that you were in the habit of eating or drinking milk or milk-based products regularly – possibly daily?

Did you find that following your Essential Diet produced marked changes in:

your weight?

any previous symptoms?

both?

Did you experience marked withdrawal symptoms?

Did you notice a craving for milk or cheese, or both?

The more *yes* answers you have, the more probable it is that you're allergic to one or more of all dairy products.

Turn to Chapter 15.

2. Did your AYAN Diary show that you were in the habit of eating grain foods (bread, cereals, cake, biscuits, pastry etc) regularly – possibly daily?

Did your Essential Diet Diary show that not eating wheat for three out of four days produced marked changes in:

your weight?

any previous symptoms?

both?

Did you experience withdrawal symptoms?

Did you crave for bread or cereals or any other grain product?

The more *yes* answers you have, the more probable it is that you're allergic to one or more or all grains.

Turn to Chapter 16.

Tea, Coffee, Alcohol

You are strongly recommended to give up all tea, coffee and alcohol during your elimination diets.

Not only do these affect the way you react to other foods, you can also be positively allergic to tea and coffee. You should appreciate too that you can be allergic to the specific constituents of your favourite alcoholic drink: to the grapes in wine, to the grains in beer and whiskey, to the apples in cider.

If you found it a real struggle to cut down on these at the start of your Essential Diet, this is a clear indication that you should cut these out – at least for the period of your diet(s). The more difficult you find it to give these (or any one of them) up, the more desirable this probably is.

However, as before, if you feel that giving all these up as well as doing your elimination diet is going to prove an impossible hurdle, then – for the time being at any rate – concentrate on your elimination diet(s), while cutting tea, coffee and alcohol down to the absolute minimum.

(Herb teas can make a welcome substitute. There's a wide range available. Experiment until you find one which appeals.)

---

3. Did your AYAN Diary show that were in the habit of eating any of the following regularly – possibly daily?

Eggs;

bacon, ham, or other pork products;

citrus fruits;

potatoes;

sugar?

135

Did you crave for any of these when you cut them down or out?

Did you notice any withdrawal symptoms which you believe have nothing to do with either grain-based foods or diary products?

Did you notice any marked changes in:

your weight?

any previous symptoms?

both?

The more *yes* answers you have, the more probable it is that you're allergic to one or more of foods in the above groups.

Turn to Chapter 17.

4. List below any of the foods or drinks *not* mentioned above which appeared at least twice a week in your AYAN Diary.

Are there any you were continuing to eat at least twice a week during your Essential Diet?

Do you particularly enjoy and look forward to any of these?

If so, it (or they) could also be causing (or contributing to) your problems.

While it's uncommon for an individual to react *only* to, say, tomatoes or apples, it's certainly not unknown.

Stone Age Diet

Some doctors choose what has become known as the Stone Age Diet as an all-round elimination diet for their allergic patients. This is based on the hypothetical primitive human diet. (See also p. 120.)

It permits all fresh meat, fish, vegetables, fruit, nuts, pulses, olive oil, spring or mineral (Malvern, Evian etc) waters; it eliminates all dairy produce, eggs, grains, sugar, tea, coffee, alcohol, and all packaged and processed foods. Some doctors restrict the diet even further, by eliminating citrus fruit; and/or beef and veal; and/or pork.

As you see, the difference – compared with your Essential Diet – is that it now cuts out at one and the same time all dairy products, grains, sugar, eggs, tea, coffee and alcohol.

The advantage in going for this straight away is that you cut out at once many potential sources of trouble. It's therefore a considerable time-saver. You can cut out, bring back and test all excluded foods within weeks.

There are also disadvantages. It demands a considerable amount of time within that period, and is difficult to combine with a working day. Because of the number of foods you're leaving out and bringing back, it's easier to carry out with professional help than without. Such a restricted diet may also be unnecessary. It's quite possible to be allergic *only* to grains or *only* to dairy products; by eliminating both at once you may be making your life pointlessly complicated.

Carrying out the Stone Age diet will certainly do you no harm from a nutritional point of view. Many people are quickly well on it – after the first few days – but some do continue to find it a struggle.

Read Categories 1 – 4 to help you decide whether to plunge in at the deep end, or whether it would make better sense to move in a different direction. If you do decide on the Stone Age diet, look first particularly at the nutritional information and alternatives in Chapters 15 and 16.

If you know in your heart that you eat a certain food unusually often or in unusually large amounts, then turn to the end of Chapter 17.

It's perfectly possible, of course, to fall into more than one category. If this is the case, then you may of course choose to follow the instructions in the relevant chapters at one and the same time. If you do, you may find the combination taxing.

If you don't, you have to bear in mind that you may then improve only gradually. But you *will* improve all the same, and you may well decide that it makes more sense to progress slowly but surely.

The French say that it's the first step that counts. You've already taken that first step. All you have to do now is keep going.

Take Care with Alternatives

If you're concerned to check up on the nutritional constituents of the foods you're eliminating, consult the Ministry of Agriculture, Fisheries and Food's Manual of Nutrition, available from any HM Stationery Office.

You'll find the following chapters suggest foods that you can use as alternatives.

137

Take care that you don't fall into the habit of using these in the same way and as often as the ones you're no longer eating. Otherwise, in the end, you could become allergic to these too. Avoid eating anything repetitively. Continue to include a wide range of foods. Vary your day-to-day diet as much as possible.

In this way your alternative foods will remain real alternatives.

CHAPTER 15

CUTTING OUT DAIRY PRODUCTS

If you suspect that you're allergic to dairy products, you're certainly not alone. More people react to dairy products than to any other group of foods.

WHY?

There are several reasons why some people are unable to tolerate dairy products. Here are just some of them.

They may have a true allergy, as defined by classical immunologists, and demonstrated by positive IgE and RAS blood tests*.

They may have a non-classic allergy (hypersensitivity), demonstrable through e.g. cytotoxic and intradermal skin testing.†

They may be reacting to toxins and pesticides transmitted through the milk.

They may be reacting to hormones.

They may be deficient in lactase – the enzyme which enables humans to digest the lactose in cow's milk. This deficiency is genetically determined: that is, you inherit it or you don't. The incidence is much higher in those of oriental, Mediterranean, black or Arab origin. In the UK it has been estimated that overall between 4% and 7% are lactase-deficient. Among white Americans, the incidence is 8%: among black Americans, 70%. 50% of Indians are deficient. Both Japanese and Greek Cypriots are 85% deficient.

Some individuals may not be able to tolerate any dairy products at all.

Others may be able to drink milk, or eat foods prepared with milk, but not eat cheese.

Others may be able to eat cheese – or perhaps only certain sorts of cheese – but not drink milk or eat any other milk products. (Cheese has undergone various chemical changes.)

*see p. 19.
†see p. 212.

CHEESE ON ITS OWN

Did your AYAN diary show that you ate cheese frequently, but used little milk?

And did your Essential Diet diary show that you disliked having to cut down on cheese, and that both eating it and not eating it were causing you problems?

Then you may if you wish start with a diet which eliminates *only* cheese.

But if you're uncertain, it's easier – and can be more time-saving in the long run – to cut out all dairy products at the same time.

This means that

you'll still be following your Essential Diet

you'll still be following your Essential Living Plan

but now in addition you'll be cutting out either *all cheese* or *all dairy products*.

All dairy products is exactly what it says.

All. This includes:

milk

cream

butter

most margarines (read the packets: almost all contain whey – which of course is milk)

all cheeses

yogurt

dried milk

anything containing any of these (be careful when you eat out)

Of course you're still not eating processed or packaged foods (are you?) because otherwise you'd need to watch out too for such disguises as 'artificial sweeteners'. Some sweeteners are milk products.

For a minimum of five days – longer if you're older: check back to p. 125 if you're uncertain – you simply don't drink or eat any of the above.

Short-term, there's nothing drastic about a diet like this from a nutritional point of view. (For long-term implications, see below.) Remember that in many parts of the world, lacking the rain that produces rich pasture-land, it's never been possible for people to rely on cow's milk or its products.

Each day you fill in your diet diary (see below): weight, how you feel, and any symptoms. Don't forget to note when they stop as well

140

as when they start.

Fill in at least five days. If you need to continue for longer than eight, use the spare sheets at the back of the book.

Remember that, if you do feel really ill during the first 24/48/72 hours, this is a very positive sign that you've identified a major cause – and possibly the *only* one – of problems.

Accept as much help and support as you can. Console yourself with the thought that you won't feel this way for long – usually not more than three to four days at most.

YOUR CHEESE/ DAIRY PRODUCTS ELIMINATION DIET DIARY

DAY ONE

BREAKFAST

MIDDAY

EVENING

EXTRAS

WEIGHT AM PM

ANY SYMPTOMS

HOW YOU FEEL

DAY TWO

BREAKFAST

MIDDAY

EVENING

EXTRAS

WEIGHT AM PM

ANY SYMPTOMS

HOW YOU FEEL

DAY THREE

BREAKFAST

MIDDAY

EVENING

EXTRAS

WEIGHT AM PM

ANY SYMPTOMS

HOW YOU FEEL

DAY FOUR

BREAKFAST

MIDDAY

EVENING

EXTRAS

WEIGHT AM PM

ANY SYMPTOMS

HOW YOU FEEL

DAY FIVE

BREAKFAST

MIDDAY

EVENING

EXTRAS

WEIGHT AM PM

ANY SYMPTOMS

HOW YOU FEEL

DAY SIX

BREAKFAST

MIDDAY

EVENING

EXTRAS

WEIGHT AM PM

ANY SYMPTOMS

HOW YOU FEEL

DAY SEVEN

BREAKFAST

MIDDAY

EVENING

EXTRAS

WEIGHT AM PM

ANY SYMPTOMS

HOW YOU FEEL

WHAT DO THE RESULTS SHOW?

On Day 6 (or later, if this makes more sense) look back at the overall picture your diary now presents.*

1. Did you notice no real change at all, apart from the inconvenience?

2. Did you observe a marked withdrawal symptoms curve, plus weight changes and diminishing symptoms?

3. Was there a change in your weight, but not in your symptoms?

4. Were there changes in your symptoms, but not in your weight?

If you were testing dairy products as a whole, and your answer to 1 was *yes*, then it's very unlikely that they have any adverse effects on you. Return to p. 134 and go on to the next possibility.

If you were testing cheese alone, and your answer to 1 was *yes*, then you could still be allergic to milk and milk-based products. Follow the guidance for eliminating dairy products as a group.

Even one *yes* answer to any of the questions 2 – 4 is a positive indication that you're reacting to cheese/dairy products. The more *yes* answers you have, the more certain you can be that this diagnosis is correct.

At this point, as explained on p. 140, you may:

1) decide simply to accept the restrictions of your cheese-free or dairy-product-free diet; or

2) experiment by reintroducing one food (or drink) at a time.

If 1), see below for advice on your new diet.

If 2), turn first to p. 130 to check up on what to do.

Then, on the sixth (or seventh to eleventh) day from the start of your elimination diet, eat a normal portion of cheese or drink a glass of milk.

Note your reactions on the chart overleaf for the next 24 hours, filling in the details under the appropriate headings. (If you have particularly severe symptoms, remember about the remedy on p. 71.)

If you feel perfectly well by midday the following day, you may have a helping of another food. If you don't feel well, wait a further 24 hours, or until you do. (Cheese in particular may sometimes produce symptoms for 48 hours, or even longer.)

Continue in the same way until you've tested everything you wish to reintroduce.

You'll find spaces for six days. You may of course not need all of

*Check with p. 147 if you wish

150

these. On the other hand, if you need to go on for longer, you'll find spare pages in the back.

JUST TO REMIND YOU . . .

After reintroduction: a change in your weight, and/or an increase in your symptoms, both indicate that you're allergic to what you're testing. A rise (or, occasionally, a fall in the pulse rate of over 10 helps to confirm this. (However, it's possible to have a weight change and/or an increase in symptoms without any accompanying pulse change. The weight change and the symptoms are more important.)

REINTRODUCTION OF CHEESE/DAIRY PRODUCTS

DAY ONE   DAY TWO   DAY THREE

TIME

WEIGHT AM PM

FOOD/DRINK

PULSE RATE
 BEFORE

AFTER 20 MINS:

40 MINS:

60 MINS

SYMPTOMS

DAY FOUR   DAY FIVE   DAY SIX

DEALING WITH A DAIRY PRODUCT-FREE DIET

By the time you've finished the reintroduction stage, you'll know which – if any – of the dairy foods you can continue to use.

For the time being, let's assume that from now on you'll be on a totally milk (milk-product)-free diet. What does this mean nutritionally; and how do you cope in the kitchen?

Of all the constituents of milk and milk products, the most significant – from a nutritional point of view – are *protein, vitamins A and B2, and calcium.**

There are many alternative sources of *protein,* both animal (meat and fish) and vegetable (pulses and nuts). Rich natural sources of *vitamin A* are liver, spinach and carrots. Among sources of *B2* are liver again, kidney, soya beans, and nuts.

So it's likely to be *calcium* which is likely to be the main cause of concern. We appreciate its importance, and we know what an excellent source milk is.

In fact, calcium is found in many other foods besides milk. Particularly good sources are green vegetables, watercress, parsley, kidney beans, tinned sardines, sesame seeds, and almonds. Carob powder (somewhat chocolatey in taste) is not only rich in calcium, but particularly useful as it can be sprinkled over a wide variety of both foods and drinks.

INSTEAD OF COW'S MILK

If you're working out a child's diet, and hence especially worried about the lack of cow's milk, then you may be able to substitute goat's milk. However, since cow and goat effectively belong to the same 'food family', then goat's milk may not be tolerable either.

Soya milk can make an effective substitute. Commercial brands contain sugar. You can make your own sugar-free soy milk.

Soy milk
3 oz (100 gms)
1½ pints (850 ml) water

*For details of other trace elements, consult the MAFF Manual of Nutrition – see p. 137.

Stir the soy flour into the water and leave to stand in a bowl for a couple of hours. Cover the bowl and place in a pan of boiling water, on top of an inverted saucer or three skewers placed in a triangle. Cover the pan, and leave to cook (make sure the water keeps at boiling point) for 20 minutes. Strain.

(Don't use the tofu-type soy milk – see below – unless you cook it thoroughly first.)

If your child can't tolerate soy milk either – which can happen – then *nut milk* is easy to make and is often very much enjoyed.

Place ground nuts (any variety) in a bowl and cover with warm water. Leave covered overnight and drain off the liquid in the morning. (If you have a blender, you can whizz the nuts/water up in this first; in which case, of course, you can also use whole instead of ground nuts.)

Quantities depend on the nuts you choose. The flavour is surprisingly strong. 2 oz per pint (50 gms per 500 ml) of water is a fair average.

Desiccated coconut can also be used like this.

Or you can try tahini milk. (Tahini is a cream made from crushed sesame seeds.) Slowly add warm water to 4 tbsp. of tahini, stirring thoroughly. It can be made more or less thick, to taste.

All these milks are rich in calcium.

INSTEAD OF CHEESE

Tofu, a curd made from soy milk, is a particularly useful alternative to cheese. It's rich in protein, and handy in the kitchen in much the same way. It can be used cold with salads, or fried in cubes, or stir-fried with mixed vegetables. Though itself bland, it easily absorbs other, stronger flavours. You can now buy it in most health food shops and many supermarkets.

It works out much cheaper if you prepare it yourself. 1 lb (500 gms) of soya beans, plus 4 tsp (20 mls) of Epsom salts, will make 1 lb (500 gms) of firm tofu. Provided you have a blender, the method's quite straightforward, although the first time you try it you'll probably find it a long-drawn out process.

Tofu

You need:

1 lb (500 gms) soya beans
4 flat tsp. (20 mls) Epsom salts
3 pints (1.75 ls) water
a blender
1 large (8 pints/5 litre) heavy based pan
1 large bowl
a piece of butter muslin (an old tea towel may do)
a piece of string
a plate or large saucer
a weight
a slotted spoon

Put the beans in a bowl. Cover with water. Leave overnight.

Next day, rinse them and put them in your blender. (If necessary, divide them into two lots.) Pour onto them, (from the 3 pints – 1.75 ls – mentioned above) approximately double their volume in water. Whizz well until smooth. Add the puree to the remaining water. Stir well.

Oil the large pan. (This helps to prevent burning.) Tie over it the muslin (or old tea towel). Pour in, bit by bit, the mixture of ground beans. Stir and push gently with a wooden spoon to force the liquid through. Finally, squeeze the cloth well. You now have a panful of soy milk.

You now have to bring this liquid to the boil. Because it contains starch, it will stick and burn readily.

So you can either bring it to the boil quickly (well, fairly quickly, because you're heating a large amount) while stirring all the time (this will take from 10-15 minutes); or leave it to come to the boil slowly over a low heat for 30-45 minutes.

Keep your eye on it once it's near boiling point. It will surge and boil over just like ordinary milk.

Once it's come to the boil, continue to simmer it for three minutes, and then remove it from the heat.

Dissolve the Epsom salts in 3 tbsp (60 mls) of warm water. Stir this solution into the bean milk.

Leave this for 5-10 minutes while you wash out the butter muslin (or tea towel) you used earlier. Rinse it well.

Drape the muslin over a colander.

By now the soy milk will have separated into curds and whey. Lift out the curds with the slotted spoon and place in the muslin-lined colander.

Rinse the curds under the cold tap.

Fold the ends of the muslin over the top of the curds. Put a plate or saucer on top, and a weight on top of that. Leave for a few hours.

This tofu will keep in the fridge for 5–7 days. If you want to keep it moist, keep it covered with water, and change the water ever other day. If you prefer it dry (because you intend to fry it, for example), just place it in a bowl covered loosely with a lid.

THE WAY AHEAD

By this stage you will either have:
1. returned to Chapter 14 to work out your next step; or
2. discovered which (if any) dairy products you can safely eat; and
3. worked out how you can cope with this change to your overall diet.

If you're now confident that you're well on the way to solving your weight (and any other problems), then you can decide whether:

you're satisfied that you've by now actually established your own A-Diet;

you feel you've got some way, but for the moment you'd rather pause and take stock;

or you feel you've made a good start, but there are still problems to solve.

If you're sure that you've successfully worked out your own A-Diet, all you need do now is stick to it, as long as you continue to lose (gain) weight, and check that any other symptoms you had have disappeared or are on the way out.

Eventually, you may even be able to cautiously reintroduce some of your now forbidden foods (but see p. 130).

You may instead feel that – although you're not completely sorted out yet – you'd rather mark time for a while before tackling another food or group of foods. That's perfectly all right.

Beef and Veal

Some people who are allergic to dairy products also react to beef and veal. If you continue to have problems, and especially if they don't seem to be connected with any of the other foods mentioned on p. 135, then it's well worth experimenting with eliminating these meats too.

But if so, remember that you *must* keep to your Essential Diet and *must* observe the restrictions. Don't complicate matters by relaxing and introducing forbidden items, or later on, if you decide to continue, you may find the whole set-up has become so confused that you risk losing your way.

But if, on the other hand, you want to tackle any remaining problems straight away, then turn back to Chapter 14, p. 128, to plan your next step.

CHAPTER 16

CUTTING OUT GRAINS

More people react to grains than to any other one group of foods, with the single exception of dairy products. Although whole grains (wholewheat, brown rice, pot barley) are excellent and highly nutritious foods in general (see p. 69), a sizeable proportion of individuals cannot tolerate them at all.

Overweight (or underweight) caused by an allergic response is probably more commonly due to grains than to any other food or group of foods. They are also implicated in such weight-connected symptoms as bloating, constipation, diarrhoea, indigestion and vomiting. Grain allergy can also be responsible for a wide range of symptoms, including, in particular, depression, tiredness, skin complaints and arthritis.

WHY?

It's strange that such staple foods should provoke reactions in a comparatively large number of individuals.

Some doctors believe, with Dr Richard Mackarness, that in evolutionary terms the human gut is not yet properly adapted to deal with the regular consumption of grains.

Some speculate that sensitive individuals may be responding to moulds in the grains, as a result of damp harvesting or storage.

Others wonder whether individuals are reacting not so much to the grains themselves, as to grains + chemicals.

Still others believe it may be the overall cumulative effect of grains (and/or grains + chemicals); that individuals become grain-sensitive because these form too large, repetitive and unbalanced a part of their overall diet.

There are certainly indications that this is at least partly the case: in the UK the grain which is the most common cause of problems is wheat, whilst in the US it is corn (maize). In the States it's almost impossible for the average American to eat a meal which does *not* contain corn: in the form either of cereal, thickener, oil, or sweetener – and of course as sweet corn or corn on the cob.

Most of the doctors concerned with this aspect of allergy are working either in Britain, certain west European countries, Australia or the States; it would be interesting to know whether rice causes similar problems in the great rice-growing areas. Certainly a few years ago the then Chinese Minister of Agriculture was urging the diversification of grain culture, saying that the Chinese were suffering from (unspecified) illnesses due to the over-consumption of rice.

CUTTING OUT GRAINS AS A GROUP

All the grain foods we commonly eat are members of one family, known in botanical language as the Gramineae. Many individuals who find that they react to one member of this large family go on to discover that they are also hypersensitive to other members.

Doctors who suspect that patients are grain-sensitive therefore normally suggest that they eliminate all the grains at once. This gives a clearer result much faster than trying to cut out one particular grain after another.

But after allergic sufferers have proved to their satisfaction that they *are* grain-sensitive, it's generally recommended that they then reintroduce them one at a time, since often they'll discover at least one or two that they can safely eat – provided that they don't eat them too regularly.

So you're now about to eliminate all grains. This means that
you'll still be following your Essential Diet
you'll still be following your Essential Living Plan
but now in addition you'll be cutting out *all* grains.

This includes everything made from:
wheat (including bran)
corn/maize (including oil)
rye
oats
rice
millet
barley

cane sugar (Tate & Lyle etc) Cane sugar comes from a plant of the same family: see also p. 182.

This means:

all breakfast cereals

all bread

all breadcrumbs

all flour or cornflour used to thicken soups or sauces

all pasta

all rice

all pastry

all variants such as couscous, semolina etc.

and naturally – as mentioned above – all cane sugar.

Of course you're still not eating processed or packaged foods (are you?) because otherwise you'd need to look out too for such disguises as 'artificial sweeteners', which could include corn syrup.

For a minimum of five days – longer if you're older: check back to p. 125 for more details – you don't eat any of the above in any form.

You won't suffer nutritionally in any way during this short period (provided, of course, you eat plenty of your Essential Diet). Remember that your faraway ancestors rarely ate grains. And they were all survivors – every single one of them.

But if you want advice *now* on alternatives and useful recipes, see below.

Meanwhile, keep your diet diary carefully. Check back to p. 127 and re-read the piece on withdrawal symptoms, so you're prepared if anything happens.

CUTTING OUT GRAINS

DAY ONE

BREAKFAST

MIDDAY

EVENING

EXTRAS

WEIGHT AM PM

ANY SYMPTOMS

HOW YOU FEEL

DAY TWO

BREAKFAST

MIDDAY

EVENING

EXTRAS

WEIGHT AM PM

ANY SYMPTOMS

HOW YOU FEEL

DAY THREE

BREAKFAST

MIDDAY

EVENING

EXTRAS

WEIGHT AM PM

ANY SYMPTOMS

HOW YOU FEEL

DAY FOUR

BREAKFAST

MIDDAY

EVENING

EXTRAS

WEIGHT AM PM

ANY SYMPTOMS

HOW YOU FEEL

DAY FIVE

BREAKFAST

MIDDAY

EVENING

EXTRAS

WEIGHT AM PM

ANY SYMPTOMS

HOW YOU FEEL

DAY SIX

BREAKFAST

MIDDAY

EVENING

EXTRAS

WEIGHT AM PM

ANY SYMPTOMS

HOW YOU FEEL

DAY SEVEN

BREAKFAST

MIDDAY

EVENING

EXTRAS

WEIGHT AM PM

ANY SYMPTOMS

HOW YOU FEEL

WHAT DO THE RESULTS SHOW?

On Day 6 (or later, if this makes more sense) look back at the overall picture your diary now presents.*

1. Did you notice no real change at all, apart from the inconvenience?

2. Did you observe a marked withdrawal symptoms curve, plus weight changes and diminishing symptoms?

3. Was there a change in your weight, but not in your symptoms?

4. Were there changes in your symptoms, but not in your weight?

If your answer to 1 was *yes*, then it's very unlikely that any grains have adverse effects on you. Return to p. 135 and go on to the next possibility.

Even one *yes* answer to any of the questions 2 – 4 is a positive indication that you're reacting to one or more grains. The more *yes* answers you have, the more certain you can be that this diagnosis is correct.

At this point, as explained on p. 160, you may decide to settle for the restrictions of your totally grain-free diet. If you're happy to stick to this, see below for some helpful advice.

It's more likely though that you'll consider it worth while experimenting by reintroducing one kind of grain at a time.

Since there is in fact a surprisingly large range – some of which you've probably only rarely if ever eaten (check with the list on p. 176), – there's a good chance that you may end up with at least one or two you can tolerate. Remember that the more grains you find you can eat, the more varied your diet can be – so if you do decide on testing, aim to include every one you can.

So, on the sixth (or seventh to eleventh) day from the start of your diet, eat a fair-sized portion of your chosen grain for that day. Use unrefined forms: wholewheat, brown rice, pot barley not pearl.

It's not easy to eat any grains entirely on their own, but try to keep the process as simple as possible. The most straightforward way (not particularly palatable, but this is only for testing), is to cook or mix each grain into a kind of porridge. It's safer to mix a pure wheat cereal with boiling water than to eat a slice of wholemeal bread (you can try this separately later), as bread also contains yeast†

*Check with p. 167 if you wish
†See p. 186.

Leave at least 48 hours between the testing of each different grain. Reactions to grains often take some time to show themselves – even as long as 72 hours. Be sure to mark the start and stop of symptoms. (If any is particularly severe, don't forget about the remedy on p. 71.)

Don't try to reintroduce the next new grain until you feel quite well and clear of symptoms.

Note your reactions on the chart overleaf for the next 24 hours or 48 hours (longer if necessary), filling in the details under the appropriate headings.

Continue in the same way until you've tested everything you wish to reintroduce.

You'll find spaces for 12 days.

Of all the foods, grains are the most troublesome, and take the longest time to sort out. (If you run out of space here, keep any extra notes safely in a notebook, or in separate pages firmly attached to this book.)

JUST TO REMIND YOU . . .

After reintroduction: a change in your weight, and/or an increase in your symptoms, both indicate that you're allergic to what you're testing. A rise (or, occasionally, a fall) in the pulse rate of over 10 helps to confirm this. (However, it's possible to have a weight change and/or an increase in symptoms without any accompanying pulse change. The weight change and the symptoms are more important.)

REINTRODUCTION OF GRAINS

DAY ONE	DAY TWO	DAY THREE

TIME

WEIGHT AM PM

FOOD/DRINK

**PULSE RATE
BEFORE**

AFTER 20 MINS:

40 MINS:

60 MINS

SYMPTOMS

DAY FOUR	DAY FIVE	DAY SIX

DAY SEVEN	DAY EIGHT	DAY NINE

TIME

WEIGHT AM PM

FOOD/DRINK

**PULSE RATE
BEFORE**

AFTER 20 MINS:

40 MINS:

60 MINS

SYMPTOMS

175

At the end of this testing period – which, as you can see, can last some time – you'll probably have discovered at least one grain you can safely eat.

If you've reacted to all of them, it's worth going on to test the more refined forms. Although these are nutritionally inferior, some people can tolerate these where they react to the whole grains. So try white rice, white bread, pearl (de-husked) barley.

If you're successful in finding a grain or grains that you can eat without reactions, don't fall into the trap of eating these as repetitively as you did the grains you're replacing. If you simply switch from having sandwiches made from wheat flour for lunch every day to sandwiches made with pure rye bread, you're likely to end up allergic to rye too.

A really varied diet is of particular importance to people with grain allergies. This often creates problems, especially in the early weeks of a totally or even partly grain-free diet.

If you – like the majority of people in this country – have relied heavily on grains in the past (cereals for breakfast, sandwiches for lunch, pies, pasta and pizzas, not to mention biscuits and cakes) you may be wondering how on earth you'll manage.

You'll find help down below. There are many alternatives which perhaps you've not yet come across.

And don't forget – even if you find you're heavily allergic at the moment, in a few months you may well be able to reintroduce them once again.

SOME IDEAS FOR LESS COMMON GRAINS

Remember that almost all grains can be found as flakes or flour, as well as whole grains. These can be used to make yeast or soda breads, scones, pancakes etc.

Pot barley can be cooked on its own like rice, or added to stews. Barley flour and barley flakes also offer a number of possibilities.

Coarse oats can be cooked in the same way. You can buy commercial oatcakes, or make your own from medium oatmeal. Porridge is a useful standby, and also contains a unique ingredient which helps to prevent diabetes.

Millet flakes also make porridge, and can be used for chapattis (see p. 93), drop scones or croquettes.

176

Rice can of course be cooked on its own. Leftover rice, chilled quickly and covered, can be safely left in the fridge four or five days to be used later as fried rice, or rice salad. There are commercially available rice biscuits (see e.g. Foodwatch list, p. 219), or you can bake them from rice flour.

Rye: you can buy pure rye bread from some delicatessens or supermarkets (but check to make sure it contains no wheat flour) – or you can bake your own. Ryvita or Ry-King both contain only rye.

To add still further variety, look at the section below.

Food Sources

Some of the foods below are available from grocers' and supermarkets, and almost all from health food shops. If you have any problems. Foodwatch (see Appendix) can supply all of these direct mail. Send a sae for price list.

WHAT IF YOU CAN EAT NO GRAINS AT ALL?

If you've discovered you're allergic to every grain you've tested, you'll be cheered to know that there are a number of alternatives. There are several foods which act (and often look like) grains, and can fill the same holes in both meals and appetites.

Here's a brief list, followed by a few thoughts of what can be done with these.

Sago: made from the trunks of the sago palm.

Tapioca: made from the root of the cassava plant.

Buckwheat: the edible seeds of a plant totally unrelated to wheat. (In fact it's a relation of rhubarb.) It's widely used in parts of Europe, particularly Eastern Europe, where it's known as kasha.

All the above are available either as whole 'grains', or as flour.

You can also use potato or chestnut flours. Other more readily available flours are chick pea (gram) flour and lentil (dhal) flour; which you'll find in any Asian grocers. (A handy and tasty bread substitute can be popadums – the Indian very thin crispy circles, as these are often made of either gram or dhal flour: but check the labels,

177

as some also contain wheat.) Soya flour is also fairly simple to find.

One other useful 'flour' is arrowroot, a very fine starch from the roots of a West Indian plant. Mixed into a paste with cold water, it can be stirred into soups, stews and sauces to thicken within a minute. Oddly enough, if you have problems finding it you may be able to buy it at your chemist's.

ALL THESE PRODUCTS ARE VERSATILE HERE ARE JUST A FEW IDEAS

Buckwheat can be left to soak overnight in unsweetened fruit juice, and then served next morning with added chopped (fresh or dried) fruit and/or nuts. It can also be cooked like rice in salted water, and served with a little butter or oil stirred in, plus onions, mushrooms, peppers etc for added interest. Buckwheat flour, used in exactly the same way as ordinary flour, makes thin lacey (Breton) pancakes.

Sago and tapioca can be cooked either in cow's milk or nut milk for an excellent breakfast cereal; or it can be simmered in the juice from cooked dried fruit – with the dried fruit chopped in afterwards. Sago and fruit, left in a greased mould and turned out when cool, sets to make a delicious cold breakfast dish for summer.

Almost all the flours can be used to make either yeast or soda breads, flat breads or scones.*

As you see, there are many alternatives to ordinary bread and cereals. The following three recipes are just a demonstration: one is for wheat-free rolls, one for a grain-free flatbread, and one for a grain-free pancake.

*Most baking powders contain a filler, usually flour. If you're allergic to wheat, write to Foodwatch for their flour-free version. Enquire too about their useful *Alternative Cookbook*.

178

3 SIMPLE RECIPES

Rye rolls
1 lb (500 gms) rye flour
2 – 2 1/2 tsp (10 – 12 mls) bicarbonate of
soda
2 – 2 1/2 tsp (10 – 12 mls) cream of tartar
1 – 2 tsp (5 – 10 mls) salt
app. 1/2 pint (300 mls) milk
1 tbsp (15 mls) oil

} the more you put
in, the lighter
the rolls, but the
stronger the taste

Stir together the flour, soda, cream of tartar, and salt. Mix the oil into the milk, and stir this steadily into the flour etc. (An ordinary large table-knife is easiest to use.) There should be enough milk to hold the mixture together, without being sticky, and to leave the bowl clean.

Rub a little oil into your hands. Knead the dough lightly to make sure it holds together, and form into a ball. Cut it across and across into eight pieces. Roll each piece between your hands into a ball. Press down lightly into a flattened roll. Place the rolls on an oiled baking tray.

Brush the tops with milk, if allowed (use your fingers if you haven't got a brush). If you like, sprinkle with sesame seeds (press down well).

Bake in a preheated oven (450 F, 230 C, Gas 8) for 15 minutes, then turn down to 400F, 200 C, Gas 6 for 10 – 15 minutes. The rolls are done when they sound hollow when tapped on the underside. Leave on a rack to cool.

Soy flat-bread
8 oz (250 gms) soy flour
1 tbsp (15 mls) oil
1/2 tsp (3 mls) salt
Water to mix.

Mix the oil briskly into a little water, and add it to the soy flour + salt, stirring with a knife. You need only just enough water to hold the flour together to make a firm dough and to leave the bowl clean. With oiled hands, form the soy dough into a fat sausage. (It can help at this stage to leave it for a while in the fridge.) Cut slices of the sausage, and with a rolling pin sprinkled with more soy flour, roll as thinly as possible. (Roll only in one direction.)

Place the pieces on an oiled tray and bake in a preheated oven (450 F, 230 C, Gas 8) for about 6 minutes. They need to be really brown, without being burnt.

Cool on a rack. Store in an airtight tin.

Buckwheat pancakes
4 oz (100 gms) buckwheat flour
1 egg
pinch of salt
approx 1/4 pint (150 mls) milk.

Make a well in the centre of the flour, add the egg, and first stir and then beat in the milk until you have a thin batter.

Heat a very little oil in a heavy or non-stick frying pan. When hot, pour in a little of the pancake mixture, tipping the pan as you do so that it flows across the pan. As soon as it bubbles and begins to look lacey, turn it over with a palette knife. Put on a hot plate under the grill, or in a low oven, while you do the others.

You can serve these pancakes with any savoury sauce, or stewed fresh or dried fruit.

(You can also make a non-milk, non-egg version of this pancake, using cider or apple juice instead of milk, and egg substitute or Bipro* instead of egg.)

So, by the end of this elimination diet, and your reintroduction of the various grains, you will have either:

1. found this was after all not relevant, and returned to Chapter 14 to work out your next step; or

2. discovered which (if any) grains you can safely eat; and worked out how you can cope with the changes to your overall diet.

If you need to go further, either check back now with Chapter 14 or move straight on to Chapter 17.

*see p. 183.

CHAPTER 17

CUTTING OUT OTHER COMMON SOURCES OF TROUBLE

Though any food *may* cause allergic reactions, some – as you know by now – are known to cause problems more frequently than others. Chief among these are:

sugar
eggs
potatoes
pork and pork products (cut meats, bacon, ham etc)
citrus fruits

If any of these came up often in your AYAN Diary, and if you've since found the restrictions on them difficult to keep to, then you should now cut it (or them) completely out of your diet.

Again, you follow your Essential Diet.
You keep to your Essential Living Plan.

If you've already found you're allergic to any grains or dairy product(s), you continue to leave it (or them) out as well.

But now, in addition, you cut out any of the above that you have reason to suspect.

If you feel you may be sensitive to more than one, then you may choose either to cut them out one at a time, or together.

Follow the instructions for elimination and reintroduction on p. 125. Keep your diaries in the pages at the end of the chapter. (If you find you're running out of space, add your observations in a notebook, or on separate pages firmly attached to this book.)

Of course, you're not exactly going to look forward to giving any of these up, especially as foods like eggs and potatoes are good nutritional standbys – and excellent natural convenience foods.

However, none of them, from a strictly nutritional point of view, contains any specific constituents which can't equally well be supplied by other foods in a balanced diet.

SUGAR

As mentioned earlier (p. 53), refined sugars should play no prominent part in the diet of anyone interested in nutrition – still less in that of anyone with weight problems.

While it's not advisable from a dietary point of view to eat more than a very modest amount of sugar (some nutritional specialists here and in the States would set this at certainly not more than 1 tbsp (20 gms) per day* – which still tots up to a good lb (500 gms) per month – some people are unable to tolerate even this amount.

They are actually allergic (hypersensitive). They may become addicted and eat it compulsively. It can give rise to many adverse symptoms, including – of course – overweight.

It's not generally appreciated that there are two kinds of ordinary granulated sugar: one processed from cane (manufactured here mainly by Tate & Lyle), and one from beet sugar (manufactured by the British Sugar Corporation).

It is perfectly possible to be allergic to one of these but not to the other. If you're allergic to grains, you're quite likely (as explained on p. x.) to be allergic to cane sugar; but perhaps able to cope with beet sugar. You may on the other hand be allergic to both beetroot and beet sugar, but able to tolerate cane sugar.

However, for all practical purposes it makes far more sense while testing to cut all ordinary commercial sugars out of your diet altogether. Eliminate them according to the general instructions on p. 125.

If sugar rated (perhaps surprisingly) high in your AYAN Diary, and you found it a great struggle even to cut it down, then you may well find that cutting it completely out of your diet is one of the most difficult things you've done.

You particularly need understanding help. Alert sympathetic friends and relatives. If you have a support group handy, be sure to call on their resources.

If you discover, by your reactions and observations, that you are indeed allergic to sugar (i.e. cane or beet or both); think well before you try to reintroduce them. You can easily do without either of them, and if you had problems withdrawing from them, reintroducing them is likely to cause you more. If you do decide on this step, possibly only to prove your allergy, introduce each sugar separately with at least 24 hours between.

*They would prefer less or none at all

There are some natural sugar substitutes available: honey (which contains some useful trace elements), date sugar and maple syrup. However, though these may be pleasant to use occasionally and in moderation, eating any of them doesn't help to wean sugar-lovers away from their passion.

If you've discovered that you're allergic, and using a substitute will really help you cope without them, then go ahead. But be particularly careful not to gradually step up your consumption of these until you're eating as much as before.

EGGS

Some people are allergic only to the yolk, others only to the white, others to both. Some can even eat eggs in some form (e.g. hard-boiled) but not another, while others react even to the merest trace left in a half-rinsed cup.

Eliminate and reintroduce for testing in the normal way. If you find you react to a whole egg, you may wish to eliminate again, and test yolk and white individually.

Eggs are good sources of (among other things) protein, iron, and vitamin D.

There are many other protein-rich foods, both animal and vegetable. Iron-rich foods include liver, kidney, dried apricots, green leafy vegetables, nuts and seeds. Vitamin D is supplied by sunlight on the skin, fish liver oils, oily fish, sunflower seeds, milk, butter and margarine. (If you can't use milk or butter, sunflower seed oil makes a useful contribution.)

So, as you see, it's not difficult to replace eggs from a nutritional point of view.

If you would like to try an alternative to help from a cooking point of view, there's a new product available called Bipro: a fine dry powder which is almost pure protein. Although processed from whey, the lactose and casein have been removed, and so it can be tolerated by some milk-allergic people. This can be used for pancakes, souffles, quiches etc.

There is also an inert (non-food) egg replacement available from Foodwatch.

Chicken

Some people allergic to eggs are also allergic to chicken. Bear this in mind as you carry on with your new diet, and if it too seems to be a possibility, eliminate it and test it in the same way.

POTATOES

Potatoes play such an essential part in the average Western daily diet that it's hard to realise that in large areas of the world they're rarely if ever eaten. And of course they were completely unknown in Britain until Sir Walter Raleigh brought them over in the sixteenth century. Although they provide a fair amount of Vitamin C, there's a good deal more in other vegetables and fruit. Instant dried potatoes, unless fortified, contain no vitamin C.

For the sensitive, potatoes can be an important cause of weight problems. As with any other food, they can also produce a wide range of symptoms, among which are skin and stomach disorders, including ulcers of various kind.

Eliminate and, if you wish, reintroduce in the normal way.

You'll miss your baked potatoes and chips if you've come to rely on them, but there are many other filling and satisfying foods available, including a whole range of grains (if tolerated), and many different pulses. You're very unlikely to be allergic to all of these, and you'll find they add variety and taste to your meals.

PORK AND PORK PRODUCTS

Although people can become allergic to any meat, more are affected by pork than by any other.* This may be partly because it's more intensively (chemically) farmed, or partly because, in its various forms, it's eaten more frequently than any other. It's perfectly possible, without realising it, to eat a pork product once or twice every day of the week.

*Few react to lamb.

184

If your original food diary showed this – or something like it – was your pattern, and that you then resented having to cut down, pork could certainly be one of your problems.

Test by eliminating all pork problems at once: pork, bacon, ham, pâtés, delicatessen meats etc.

There is no nutritional problem in cutting out all pork products and simply not eating any of them again.

However, because it's possible to be allergic *only* to bacon, or to ham, or to sausages, or to particular delicatessen meats, you may if you wish experiment with introducing each of these separately, at intervals of at least 24 hours, as explained on p. 130.

If you do subsequently discover a version of pork you can safely eat, then be sure not to overdo it. Treat it with caution. Don't eat it more than twice a week at most – preferably less.

CITRUS FRUITS

It seems especially odd to have citrus fruits featuring well up in the list of foods that some people cannot eat.

It has been suggested – as mentioned earlier – that citrus fruits are such a new part of the diet of European peoples that that we're still ill-adapted to eating them in any quantity. It's only very recently indeed that they've become available in such quantities and right through the year. Prepared pure juices, which mean that people can drink the equivalent of several fruits at one go, may perhaps also contribute to over-consumption.

There is also, of course, the fact that all citrus crops grown commercially for export are heavily treated by chemicals at various stages.

Though, nonetheless, most can still eat them safely, some individuals can't. The one which provokes most reactions is the orange. Grapefruit, lemon, and other varieties come some way after.

Test by eliminating all the citrus fruits together, and reintroducing them – if you decide to – one at a time.

Though citrus fruits may indeed be excellent sources of vitamin C, there are many others: most fresh fruits and vegetables, particularly local vegetables in season, and especially when eaten raw.

CUTTING OUT LESS COMMON FOODS

There is no food (or drink) which can be guaranteed to cause no allergic reactions in anyone. Although all those mentioned so far are the ones which most frequently cause allergic reactions in people on typical Western diets, there are several others which also crop up relatively often.

These include:

tomatoes
bananas
onions
peanuts
fish
mushrooms
yeast

Yeast and mushrooms are closely connected. Those who are allergic to one are often allergic to the other. If you discover that you can't eat yeast, this of course means cutting out bread etc made with yeast, all alcohol, yeast extract, and of course yeast tablets.

Any other single food, however unlikely, can also be involved: even such apparently totally innocuous foods as lettuce, cabbage, carrots, or apples.

Again, the clue that any food (or drink) may be affecting you can be seen in how often you used to have it (as shown in your AYAN Diary); and how often you continued to have it, or how much you missed not having it, during the period of your Essential Diet.

The more you enjoyed it, the more frequently you ate/drank it, the greater the chance that whatever-it-is has been contributing to your problems.

Look searchingly through your records. Remember that having something even as infrequently as twice a week could be enough to make it suspect.

If you spot a likely candidate, follow again exactly the same procedure.

If you do discover you're allergic to any similar foods to those suggested above, leaving them out altogether isn't going to present any real nutritional problems. The main difficulty is likely to be social – trying to avoid the ever-present tomato or mushroom, for example, when eating out.

However, remember that you may well, before too long, be able to try these out again (see p. 130).

Some of these foods are more obviously directly connected with weight problems than others. However, what's important is not only the effect of the foods themselves, but the fact that an actual allergy to any one of them can affect the whole way the body functions. So it's wise to continue keeping an eye open for anything in the future you find yourself beginning to eat or drink in unaccustomed quantities.

Tap Water

Among the more apparently bizarre causes of allergic problems is *tap water*.

Because it never enters most people's head to suspect that this could be the case, when it does happen it can go on creating problems for months or years. One sign that this could be the case is the drinking of large amounts of water* which can lead to sudden unexplained weight gains (and losses).

Some people are reacting to the chlorine in the water. When this is the case the use of a filter will do the trick. If you suspect this possibility, try using the Brita* water jug, and see if there's any improvement.

Others, though, may be reacting to any of a whole range of minerals or heavy metals. If you still suspect water, and de-chlorinating it isn't the answer, then switch to pure mineral waters (e.g. Malvern, Evian), at least for a testing period.

(Steaming vegetables, rather than simmering them, is a more economical way of using expensive waters.)

*also of course a sign of diabetes,
*See Appendix

YOUR ELIMINATION DIARY

DAY ONE

BREAKFAST

MIDDAY

EVENING

EXTRAS

WEIGHT AM PM

ANY SYMPTOMS

HOW YOU FEEL

DAY TWO

BREAKFAST

MIDDAY

EVENING

EXTRAS

WEIGHT AM PM

ANY SYMPTOMS

HOW YOU FEEL

DAY THREE

BREAKFAST

MIDDAY

EVENING

EXTRAS

WEIGHT AM PM

ANY SYMPTOMS

HOW YOU FEEL

DAY FOUR

BREAKFAST

MIDDAY

EVENING

EXTRAS

WEIGHT AM PM

ANY SYMPTOMS

HOW YOU FEEL

DAY FIVE

BREAKFAST

MIDDAY

EVENING

EXTRAS

WEIGHT AM PM

ANY SYMPTOMS

HOW YOU FEEL

DAY SIX

BREAKFAST

MIDDAY

EVENING

EXTRAS

WEIGHT AM PM

ANY SYMPTOMS

HOW YOU FEEL

DAY SEVEN

BREAKFAST

MIDDAY

EVENING

EXTRAS

WEIGHT AM PM

ANY SYMPTOMS

HOW YOU FEEL

DAY EIGHT

BREAKFAST

MIDDAY

EVENING

EXTRAS

WEIGHT AM PM

ANY SYMPTOMS

HOW YOU FEEL

YOUR REINTRODUCTION DIARY

DAY ONE	DAY TWO	DAY THREE

TIME

WEIGHT AM PM

FOOD/DRINK

PULSE RATE
BEFORE

AFTER 20 MINS:

40 MINS:

60 MINS

SYMPTOMS

DAY FOUR	DAY FIVE	DAY SIX

CHAPTER 18

CHEMICALS AND OTHER HAZARDS

If you answered *yes* to all four questions 15–18, then you're one of the people for whom this chapter should have perhaps come first of all. Even if you only answered *yes* to one, that one yes could - without your ever suspecting it - play a significant part in your weight problems and your previous diet failures.

HERE'S WHY

Exposure to chemicals affects the way people's bodies behave.

Some will be affected more, some less, because individual's reactions to chemicals vary very considerably.

Some chemicals are recognised as being universally dangerous in sufficient quantities: the old coal gas is a good example. Breathe in enough of it, and any individual - no matter what his or her individual susceptibility might be - will die. North Sea gas is not toxic in the same way. Nonetheless, certain individuals will react to it. Some are so exquisitely sensitive that even the most minute trace - so small that it won't even register on conventional equipment - will produce harmful reactions.

Other chemicals are not thought of as being dangerous in the same way as coal gas was known to be. They're considered 'safe': or, at least, safe in the quantities in which most people are supposed to encounter them.

In actual fact, it is not easy to either establish or keep within universally 'safe' limits. There are four main reasons.

1. Individual chemical susceptibility varies so considerably.*

2. Even where hypothetically safe limits are set, there's often insufficient incentive or supervision to ensure they are observed.

*See *Biochemical Individuality*, Dr Roger Williams, University of Texas Press, 1956

3. Since many chemicals remain in the body, individuals may accumulate doses which may be theoretically 'safe' but which cumulatively are potentially harmful.

4. No allowance is made for the fact that chemicals may interreact and together present different hazards than either singly.

These chemicals may affect the body in various ways. One of these may be to damage the immune system, with the result that it may accelerate the development of food allergies.

In practice, what this means is that some people develop food allergies *because* they're affected by chemicals. The chemical reactions and food reactions go together. When an individual becomes allergic to both foods and chemicals it isn't easy to disentangle the effects of each.

Fortunately, there are steps individuals can take to protect themselves

A good diet of fresh, safe foods helps to counteract the effects of chemicals; removing, or cutting down on, the chemicals helps to make food-allergic individuals less hypersensitive.

Chapters 1 – 16 are primarily concerned with the food side.

This looks, briefly, at certain chemicals – and their possible effect on you and your diet.

MEDICALLY-PRESCRIBED OR OVER-THE-COUNTER DRUGS

All drugs, even the most apparently innocuous, have effects other than those they're intended to. The side-effects of many are known to include changes in the gut and on the central nervous system, and are known to be linked with both weight gains or losses and on the psychological reactions of those who take them. Drugs may help to bring about, not only the development of food allergies, but the perversion of appetite which frequently accompanies them. They may also, of course, produce actual allergic reactions.

Over-the-counter drugs are, by definition, ones that are considered safe enough to be taken without medical advice or supervision. Yet any of these, if powerful enough to affect the body in one way, is powerful enough also to affect it in another. One of the most common, aspirin, is known to cause allergic reactions in a proportion of takers.

If you're in the habit of taking any over-the-counter drug with any regularity, then it makes sense to cut it/them out before starting on any diet proper. By all means continue with anything you habitually take while you fill in your first food (As You Are Now) diary. This will help to show you what effect, if any, they're having.

But before you start on your Essential Diet (p. 65), stop taking them.

In any case, you may very well find that the symptoms for which you've been taking them will begin to diminish or disappear.

Prescribed drugs should, for present purposes, be divided into the absolutely essential, and others.

There are few actual life-savers. You will know if you are on one of these.

There exist a whole range of other drugs which relieve pain or suppress symptoms, but are not strictly speaking unavoidable (though removal of them may, as a result of withdrawal symptoms, produce a threatening situation).

If you have been regularly taking drugs in the second group, then it is suggested that you discuss with your GP the possibility of stopping, or at least gradually reducing, these while you work your way towards your A-Diet. (Again, you may, in any case, discover that the symptoms for which these were prescribed are among those actually caused by food allergies.)

Tranquillisers, anti-depressants and sleeping-pills are all among those most frequently prescribed for food-allergic patients, and which actually contribute to the creation and maintenance of the food allergies causing the symptoms for which they are prescribed. Pharmaceutically speaking, with rare exceptions, none of these should be prescribed for other than very short periods: it is suggested that three weeks should be considered the maximum. If you've been taking them longer than this, then the strong probability is that they are now not only ineffective but damaging.

Again, ask your GP for help. It is very unwise simply to stop taking them, as you are likely to suffer acute withdrawal symptoms. It's necessary to cut them down gradually.

If your GP is unhelpful, or you need more support, get in touch with Release and/or TRANX.*

If you face great problems in cutting drugs down or out, then go on to the next stage anyway. Follow the Essential Diet, and the Essential

*See Appendix.

200

Living Plan (p. 97), but be gentle with yourself. If you find it too hard to observe all the restrictions on cutting down on bread, cheese and sugar, for example, then go easy on these. But be sure to cut out the processed foods (which also contain chemicals); and eat plenty of fresh vegetables and fruit, particularly raw. (These provide essential vitamins of which your drugs have probably been depriving you.)

THE PILL

The Pill is commonly associated in people's minds with weight gains. (In fact, increased weight is one of the most common reasons for women to stop taking it.) It's less widely known that it can also cause gradual weight loss.

It also destroys the effect of certain vitamins, changes the mineral balance, and affects such essentials as liver function; it's now also believed, by specialists both here and abroad, to cause long-term damage to the immune system.*

This means that it can cause, or help to cause, food allergies.

Since few overweight people continue to take the Pill, the chances are that, if you did, you no longer do. However, if you indeed *are* on the Pill, you're recommended to stop before starting on your Essential Diet. (And if you were on the Pill, but no longer are, it could help to explain why you could have become food allergic.)

And why you still are. Because once you stop taking the Pill – or indeed any other drug – your body doesn't immediately snap back to its pre-Pill (or pre-drug) state. It takes time for it to get rid of chemicals: and their effects.

CHEMICALS IN YOUR ENVIRONMENT

Exposure to chemicals where you work or live or actually in your home can also affect you. And, again, one of the effects may be damage to the immune system, and hence an increased likelihood of developing food allergies.

Among the many possible hazards are:

*See *The Bitter Pill* by Ellen Grant, Corgi, 1986

agricultural sprays
treatment for woodwork and dry rot
foam insulation
waste fumes from factories
diesel and petrol fumes
household gas
aerosols
paint fumes
insecticides
disinfectants
bleach
dry-cleaning fluids
carbonless carbon
fluids used in copying machines
air conditioning
air fresheners
deodorants
clothes conditioners
felt-tipped pens
and many others.

As explained above, not everyone will be affected in the same way. Some individuals will react to very much smaller amounts than others. Also, while chemicals affect the way the body handles food, the kind of food being eaten also affects the way the body copes with chemicals. Someone on a varied diet of fresh foods is better equipped to minimise the danger caused by chemicals. And the more you cut down on your exposure to chemicals, the less effect overall they will have on you.

So there are ways in which you can help yourself.

AT HOME

Do away with all unnecessary chemicals- such as aerosols and insect sprays – altogether.

Use the smallest quantities possible of the chemicals that you do use.

Consider using non-chemical alternatives. For example, there are cleaners based on coconut oils and not on petroleum-based detergents.*

When you use any strongly-smelling chemical in the house, such as paint or varnish, get as much through ventilation as possible.

AT WORK

If others feel the same way as you, make a concerted attempt to improve conditions. Seek union involvement.

Press for strongly smelling chemicals to be shut away when not used.

Press for adequate ventilation.

Press for air-conditioning systems to be regularly checked.

Press for smoke free zones.

CHEMICALS IN FOODS

ADDITIVES

If your regular diet has included many processed foods and soft drinks, or certain sorts of takeaways, then it will certainly have included many additives. Not all of these are synthetics. Some – for example, sugar, certain natural colourings – are not. But many (most) are.

The Soil Association's *Look at the Label Again* (see p. 219) and *E for Additives* (M. Hanssen, Thorsons 1984) will give you all the details.

Meanwhile, here's some brief information to be going on with.

Some of the most suspect additives are chemical colourings added purely for cosmetic reasons. Several of these are azo dyes, close relations (chemically speaking) of aspirin – so anyone sensitive to aspirin should be particularly on the look out for these.

*Incidentally, some people are allergic to the actual detergent base of most shampoos; for these, it is the shampoo itself which causes their 'dry scalp'.)

Two of the most common are tartrazine (E102) an orangey-yellow, and amaranth (E 123), a red. Tartrazine is found in a whole range of food products and drinks, such as breadcrumbs, orange squash, desserts, soups, vegetables etc. Another (banned abroad) is Brown FK, used for kippers and smoked fish. Tartrazine and amaranth are both often present – but unidentified – in medicines, tablets and vitamin pills.

Monosodium glutamate (MSG) – the cause of the so-called Chinese Restaurant Syndrome – is also found in the majority of processed foods.

Among the most suspect preservatives are sulphur dioxide (E220–227), nitrites and nitrate (E249–252), and BHA and BHT (E320 and E321). The UK Food Standards Committee has twice recommended that BHT should be banned.

Artificial flavourings account for 3,000 out of the estimated 3,500 additives in use. Their constituents are considered commercial secrets, they are not specifically regulated, and few have been tested for safety. Watch out for the key word 'flavour', which shows that the source is mainly or entirely synthetic.

While occasional exposure to a few additives may do little harm to most, some individuals are sensitive even to infinitesimal amounts. Others become increasingly sensitive as their intake increases. Still others will react to *combinations* of the different chemicals.

Because chemical additives in food are known to contribute to the food allergy problem, and because they are the most easily avoided of all chemicals (all you have to do is neither buy them or eat them), your Essential Diet, and hence your ultimate A-Diet, is planned to avoid them completely. (Later, it may be possible to modify this: see p. 130.)

PESTICIDES, HERBICIDES ETC

Foods not only have chemicals deliberately added. Many arrive in the shops already carrying within them and on them the traces of the chemicals with which they have been treated during the whole growing process.

Such chemicals present in foods present a different, hidden hazard. Food grown organically (that is, naturally and without chemicals) is hard to find, and, not suprisingly, more expensive. However, some supermarkets now regularly supply small amounts.

For some hypersensitive individuals there is no option: they can only tolerate organically grown food. For the rest of us with diet problems, it makes sense to grow food naturally if at all possible, to buy it when we can, and otherwise to concentrate on avoiding unnecessary chemicals elsewhere.

SMOKING

Some people continue smoking because they think they'll put on weight if they stop – yet you probably know any number of overweight people who also smoke.

Apart from the other known health hazards of cigarettes, smoking – in introducing chemicals into the body – also damages the immune system. (In fact smoking is one of *the* major causes of migraines and severe headaches.)

Hence smokers are more likely then non-smokers to acquire food allergies.

If you do smoke, it would certainly be wiser to stop – ideally, before you start on your Essential Diet; if not then, before you go on to any of the elimination diets. Although on the one hand you may dread the thought of coping both with no cigarettes and a new diet, in practice you may well find that this takes the edge off your craving for nicotine.

If, though, you suffer from bad withdrawal symptoms (see also p. x.), remember that the first few days are the worst. They won't last, and you will get over it. (If this turns into a problem on its own, write to Ash* for their advice and fact-sheets.)

Moulds

Hardly chemicals, not precisely pollutants: but moulds of all kinds can cause troublesome reactions in just the same way.

Keep rooms well aired. Don't store old sheets or rags in damp cupboards. Keep condensation at bay by using tubs of absorbent crystals. Wash mould away from walls and ceilings with a dilute solution of bleach (a lesser of two evils) and ventilate the room well afterwards.

*See Appendix

Doctors who work in the field of food and chemical allergies have arrived at the concept of 'total burden' or 'total overload' to describe how likely any individual is to become or remain allergic. The 'total burden' is made up of all the possible factors which can induce food allergy.

Among all these factors, chemicals play an important and ever-increasing role. If you remove as many chemical hazards as you can, you're reducing the burden on your body. You may notice no difference in the extreme short term, but you're very likely to in the long run. Some people even find that, once their exposure to chemicals is reduced or removed, their food allergies also diminish or disappear. Even if only as a safety precaution, it is well worth consciously cutting out all chemicals you can easily dispense with.

CHAPTER 19

SOME USEFUL EXTRAS

FOOD FAMILIES

As you've seen in earlier chapters, people who are allergic to one food are often (but certainly not always) allergic to others in the same family – because these foods are in fact very similar.

Here, just to put you on your guard, are some of the most frequently eaten fruit-and-vegetable foods divided into their botanical families.

Carrot family
carrot
celeriac
celery
coriander
cumin
fennel
lovage
parsley
parsnip

Composite family
chicory
globe artichoke
Jerusalem artichoke
lettuce
safflower (oil)
salsify
sunflower (and oil)

Goosefoot family
beet
chard

spinach
sugar beet (and therefore beet sugar)

Gourd family
cucumber
courgette (zucchino)
marrow
melon
pumpkin
watermelon

Grape family
grape (and all alcoholic grape products)
currants, raisins and sultanas
wine vinegar

Lily family
asparagus
chives
garlic
leek
onion

Mustard family
broccoli
Brussels sprouts (and sprout tops)
cabbage
cauliflower
Chinese leaves
curly kale
kohlrabi
radish
swede
turnip (and turnip tops)
watercress

Potato family
aubergine (eggplant)
pepper (red and green); also paprika
potato

tobacco
tomato

Rose family
Group 1
  apple (therefore cider and cider vinegar)
  pear (thus perry)
Group 2
  almond
  apricot
  cherry
  peach (and nectarine)
  plum (prune)
Group 3
  blackberry
  loganberry
  raspberry
  strawberry

Legume family
alfalfa
beans (all beans, including bean sprouts)
carob
pea (including chickpea – garbanzo)
peanut (and peanut oil)
soya beans and all soy products (including oil)

Rue (Citrus) family
grapefruit
lemon
lime
orange
tangerine (and all similar versions)

If you've discovered that you're allergic to any of the above, keep a sharp lookout for any unusual reactions to any others in the same group.

CANDIDIASIS

Doctors are increasingly finding that some patients with food allergies are also suffering from candida albicans: an overgrowth of otherwise harmless organisms in the gut.

For women, the significant clues that this may be the case are:
cystitis
gynaecological and period problems
a hysterectomy
being a Pill-taker, or an ex-Pill-taker
having been prescribed a course of steroids
thrush
any vaginal discharge, not necessarily diagnosed as thrush

For men, the relevant clues are:
all prostatic problems.

For both, it's significant if there has been any past illness (particularly sore throats or acne) for which antibiotics have been prescribed; particularly if that antibiotic was Tetracycline.

If any of the above applies to you, and you've made less than totally satisfactory progress, then visit your GP and ask for his advice. (The normal treatment is a course of Nystatin.) Or, if you prefer, you may visit a homeopath and be treated for this homeopathically; or you may use acidophilus powder. It's also important to go on a totally yeast-free diet and to eat foods (natural yogurt, olive oil, or garlic) which attack the candida.*

*To know more about this in detail, read *The Yeast Connection*, by William G. Crook, Professional Books; or *Candida Albicans* by Leon Chartow, Thorsons.

VITAMIN AND MINERAL SUPPLEMENTS

It's not a good idea to self-dose on vitamins or minerals; ideally, you need a doctor with specialist experience to be able to advise you.

Hair analysis will show certain mineral deficiencies and high toxic metal levels, but again it needs a skilled interpreter to know what the readings mean.

Lacking any such help, the only supplements which can be sensibly recommended are the following.

Vitamin C This is the only vitamin the human body doesn't manufacture for itself. Even on a high-fruit, high-vegetable diet it's possible – especially in times of stress or illness – to run short of this. Some vitamin C is destroyed by chemical farming methods. Some disappears en route from farm to the kitchen. More is destroyed by cooking.

It's perfectly safe to take Vitamin C supplements daily. It is in any case a water-soluble vitamin, and any excess (though you would have to take a great deal in a very short time for there to be any) would simply be washed out of the body.

Multivitamin supplement Provided you don't exceed the stated dose, you can safely use a multivitamin supplement. It can be particularly useful if you're eliminating a whole group of foods, such as grains or dairy products.

Since some commercial vitamins contain (undisclosed) colourings, ask your pharmacist for information about this, or else buy your vitamins from a knowledgeable health food shop or a similar direct mail source.

Evening primrose oil + vitamin E This can be especially beneficial for women during their fertile years (from puberty to the menopause), particularly for those who previously suffered (or still suffer) from premenstrual tension. It may in some cases be prescribable through the NHS.

Zinc Some people with symptoms of food allergy are found to be deficient in zinc. British diets tend to be low in zinc-rich foods. Women who are or have been on the Pill may also have low zinc levels as this alters the zinc/copper ratio in the body. A zinc deficiency alters the way in which the body behaves.*

---

*Zinc supplements have been shown to help in cases of both bingeing and anorexia.

It may be helpful to take a zinc supplement (available through health shops and certain chemists), particularly during or after elimination diets. Be careful not to exceed the stated quantity.

ALLERGY TESTS AND POSITIVE INTERVENTION TREATMENT

Allergy tests available through the NHS are of limited use. IgE and RAS tests will only pick up allergies as defined by classical immunologists (see p. 19). Skin prick tests, though reasonably accurate for inhalants (dust, pollen etc) are so inaccurate for foods as to be meaningless.

There do exist other methods for testing and diagnosis, but available at present only from private clinics.

Those available include:
intradermal skin testing
cytotoxic testing
kynesiology
electrical measurements
skin, sweat and urine tests.

The above tests can be very helpful, but *only* in the hands of an experienced practitioner who is able to interpret and advise.*

All doctors treating food allergies recommend removing harmful foods as the basic and most important course.

However, this does present problems, particularly for those who react to many different foods, or who are forced frequently to eat away from home. For allergic individuals with such difficulties, there are actual treatments available.

These take two basic forms.

1. *Neutralisation.* Infinitely minute dilutions of harmful foods are prescribed in the form either of drops or injections, to be taken one or more times per day.

2. *Enzyme Potentiated Desensitization (EPD)* A vaccination of enzyme-treated extracts of foods is given at long intervals: at first a few times each year, and then less frequently.

Consultations involving either testing or treatment are at present available only privately.

*For further information, see *The Allergy Connection*.

It is possible – provided a GP accepts the diagnosis and proposed treatment – for the drops (or injections) needed for neutralisation to be re-prescribed by the GP provided under the NHS.

EPD is still available only privately.

In-patient diagnosis and treatment is also available – again only privately – in two specialist clinics: one in the north and one in the south of England.

AAA, the NSRA and the HCSG may be able to advise you (see p. 219) concerning the testing and treatments mentioned above.

CHAPTER 20

AND THE FUTURE?

Once you've established your A-Diet, it's only sense – as suggested earlier – to keep to it for several months. As long as you continue to lose (gain) weight, and you're fit, well, and happy, then you probably won't want to risk changes. (And don't forget the exercise!)

At some point, though, you'll probably want to discover whether you're still allergic to the foods and drinks you've cut out – or whether you can actually start including them again quite happily.

As you'll appreciate by now, the only way you can find this out is by reintroducing and testing again.

Here's what to do.

Make sure you have a remedy handy in case you get a bad reaction (see p. 71).

On the chosen day, have a reasonable portion of whatever-it-is for breakfast. If you have no reaction, have it again as part of your lunch. If still no reaction, have it again in the evening. Note any changes in your weight or pulse rate, or any new symptoms, over the next 48–72 hours.

After your previous months of abstinence, you may expect *one of three possibilities*.

You may still have your former allergy, and it seems not at all diminished. In this case, you'll react very strongly. (This is relatively unusual.)

You may have lost the allergy completely, and you won't react at all.

Or you may fit somewhere in between – you've become more tolerant, and react only slightly.

It's not possible to predict what will happen in any particular case. The only possible clue is that the lighter your total burden has now become (maybe you're a happier person; you're working in a new job where you're less exposed to chemicals; you've stopped smoking), the less likely you are to react; and the longer you leave it before you try, the safer you're likely to find it.

If you pass your test with a clean bill, then you can feel free to start eating whatever-it-is again – provided, needless to say, that you use it only in moderation. If you start relaxing to the extent that you again eat it frequently – let alone daily – then you certainly risk the return of your previous problems.

If you do show any changes in weight, pulse rate or symptoms, then leave out the suspect item for at least another three months.

As time goes by, you may also experiment with relaxing the other restrictions. Always remain on your guard. If you do start to put on/lose weight, or begin to get headaches or indigestion or feel unwell in any way: then stop. Go back to your A-Diet.

And, as a result of the latest trends, you can begin to look once more at the possibilities of – at least occasionally – making use of prepared foods. Several of the supermarkets are now introducing foods at least without colourings, and sometimes without additives altogether. Some tinned vegetables too – useful as stand-bys – are also now available without either colourings or sugar.

The A-Diet isn't fixed for ever. It may change as you, your life and your circumstances change. But from now on you know the secret – which is no secret: and you can go on to adapt it so that it suits you, not just now, but through all the months and years to come.

P.S. WHERE YOU ARE NOW

Your totally unsafe foods/drinks are:..

....

....

Your suspect foods/drinks are..

Symptoms you no longer have...

Symptoms (if any) you still have..

Drugs you no longer take...

Drugs you still take (if any)..

Chemicals you're no longer exposed to...

Weight

Measurements

    Chest   Upper arms

    Neck   Upper thighs

    Waist   Wrists

    Hips   Ankles

How your skin looks

Your present state of health

How you feel

Any other comments

P.P.S

If by now you've noticed marked improvements, but your weight problems are still not completely solved, and you still have troublesome symptoms, then you're strongly recommended to seek further advice.

Certain individuals may have particularly delayed reactions to certain foods; and/or may be heavily deficient in certain vitamins and minerals as the result of severe past illnesses; and/or have been actively poisoned or otherwise damaged by over-exposure to chemicals. It is also perfectly possible, of course, that a more mundane diagnosis has been overlooked.

Check again with your GP that there is nothing obviously wrong; perhaps read some of the books recommended in the text of the A-Diet and in the Appendix; and/or consider further tests or consulting a specialist.

Look back again to pp. 102 and 212 on where to look for help.

As an allergic, previously overweight mother recently put it: 'It's been a struggle, but so well worth persevering, even though it took much longer than I expected. I only wish I'd known about this when my first daughter was born. I'm sure I could have sorted myself out then in half the time, and saved myself so much misery.

'I'm going to try to make sure that from now on none of my family ever goes through what I had to. But at any rate that's all behind me now – and I'm quite determined to make up for all those wasted years!'

APPENDIX

The following charities will supply information on various aspects of allergy. Members receive regular newsletters, advice on helpful contacts, addresses of local support groups, and other practical assistance.

Action Against Allergy, 43 The Downs, London SW20 8HG

National Society for Research into Allergy, PO Box 45, Hinckley, Leicestershire LE10 1JY

Hyperactive Children's Support Group, 59 Meadowside, Angmering, Littlehampton, West Sussex BN16 4BW

The Homoeopathic Development Foundation, 19a Cavendish Square, London W1M 9AD, gives information on homoeopathy and details of local homoeopaths.

Release, 1 Elgin Avenue, London W9, will give help and information on all drugs.

Tranx, 17 Peel Road, Harrow, Middlesex HA3 7QX, helps those on tranquillisers or sleeping-pills.

The McCarrison Society, 76 Harley Street, London W1N 1AE, is concerned to study the relationship between nutrition and health; it also publishes the work of Sir Robert McCarrison.

The Henry Doubleday Research Association, Ryton on Dunsmore, Coventry CV8 3LG, and *The Soil Association*, Walnut Tree Manor, Stowmarket, Suffolk, will advise on growing organic foods. They also have constantly updated lists of sources of organic produce.

Foodwatch, Butts Pond Industrial Estate, Sturminster Newton, Dorset DT10 1AZ, provides mail order a wide range of additive-free basic foodstuffs.

Larkhall Laboratories, 225 Putney Bridge Road, London SW15, supplies mail order vitamins and minerals, and also various food substitutes.

SOME USEFUL BOOKS

(Books detailed in the text are omitted here)

Most of these books should be available in any bookshop. Wholefood (24 Paddington Street, London W1) and Junkantique (43 The Downs, London SW20 8HG) both stock a wide range dealing with all aspects of health: catalogues are available on request with sae. Books published by Thorsons are also available direct from their mail order department: Denington Estate, Wellingborough, Northants NN8 2RQ.

The Right Way to Eat, Miriam Polunin (J.M. Dent/Europa, 1984)

Health on Your Plate, Janet Pleshette (Hamlyn Paperbacks, 1983)

The Whole Health Manual, Patrick Holford (Thorsons, 1983)

The Vitamins Explained Simply, Leonard Mervyn (Thorsons, 1984)

The Organic Food Guide, ed. by Alan Gear (Henry Doubleday Research Association, 1983)

Food Additives, Erik Millston (Thorsons, 1986)

E for Additives Supermarket Shopping Guide, ed. by Maurice Hanssen (Thorsons, 1986)

Not All in the Mind, Richard Mackarness (Pan, 1976)

Chemical Victims, Richard Mackarness (Pan, 1980)

Life Without Tranquillisers, Vernon Coleman (Corgi, 1986)

Tracking Down Hidden Food Allergies, W.G. Crook (Professional Books, 1980)

Allergies Your Hidden Enemy, Theron G. Randolph and Ralph W. Moss (Turnstone Press, 1981)

The Cookery Year (Reader's Digest Association Ltd., 1973)

Delia Smith's Complete Cookery Course, BBC Publications.

Gardening without Chemicals, Jack Temple (Thorsons, 1983)

A FEW USEFUL EXTRAS

The Brita water jug, manufactured by Brita UK Ltd., Ashley Road, Walton-on-Thames, Surrey, is available at most health food shops and chemists.

For information about Bipro, write to Earthlore Ltd., Ross-on-Wye, Herts HR9 6BX.

A useful, dividable, heavy-duty shopping trolley is available from JanieJak Designs, Beaumont House, Herongate, Rickmansworth, Herts WD3 5BP.

NON FICTION AVAILABLE
FROM PATHWAY

THE PRICES SHOWN BELOW WERE CORRECT AT THE TIME OF GOING TO
PRESS. HOWEVER TRANSWORLD PUBLISHERS RESERVE THE RIGHT TO
SHOW NEW RETAIL PRICES ON COVERS WHICH MAY DIFFER FROM THOSE
PREVIOUSLY ADVERTISED IN THE TEXT OR ELSEWHERE.

☐ 17275 1	Making Love During Pregnancy	*Elizabeth Bing & Libby Colman*	£3.50
☐ 12815 5	The Headache and Migraine Book	*J. N. Blau*	£3.50
☐ 12734 5	The Patient's Companion	*Vernon Coleman*	£3.95
☐ 99238 0	Addicts and Addictions	*Vernon Coleman*	£3.50
☐ 17356 1	Running Without Fear	*Kenneth Cooper*	£3.95
☐ 12798 1	The Bitter Pill	*Dr. Ellen Grant*	£3.50
☐ 99242 9	Judith Hann's Total Health Plan	*Judith Hann*	£2.95
☐ 99246 1	Coming To Terms	*Roberta Israeloff*	£3.50
☐ 17274 3	Recipes For Diabetics	*Billie Little & Penny L. Thorup*	£3.95
☐ 17273 5	The Herb Book	*Ed. John Lust*	£4.95
☐ 99244 5	Homeopathic Medicine At Home	*Maesimund B. Panos & Jane Heimlich*	£4.95
☐ 12829 5	The A For Allergy Diet	*Barbara Paterson*	£2.95
☐ 12822 8	New Ways To Lower Your Blood Pressure	*Claire Safran*	£3.50
☐ 13002 8	Stress Without Distress	*Hans Selye*	£2.95
☐ 17272 7	Getting Well Again	*Carl & Stephanie Simonton*	£3.95

All these books are available at your bookshop or newsagent, or can be ordered direct from the publisher. Just tick the titles you want and fill in the form below.

Transworld Publishers, Cash Sales Department, 61–63 Uxbridge Road, Ealing, London,
W5 5SA

Please send a cheque or postal order, not cash. All cheques and postal orders must be in £
sterling and made payable to Transworld Publishers Ltd.
Please allow cost of book(s) plus the following for postage and packing:

U.K./Republic of Ireland Customers:
Orders in excess of £5; no charge
Orders under £5; add 50p

Overseas Customers:
All orders; add £1.50

NAME (Block Letters) ....

ADDRESS ....

....